UNDERSTANDING THE POWER OF THE X FACTOR

Marianna Haun

The Russell Meerdink Company, Ltd.
Neenah, WI 54956

Library of Congress Cataloging-in-Publication Data

Haun, Marianna, 1945-

Understanding the power of the X factor/Marianna Haun.

p. cm.

ISBN 0-929346-68-8

1. Race horses—Genetics. 2. Heart—Size. 3. X chromosome.
4. Sex-linkage (Genetics). 5. Race horses—Speed. I. Title.

SF338 .H379 2001
636.1'221—dc21

2001048508

Cover design: Bosetti Production Art & Design
Book layout and design: Robin Driessen

Published by

The Russell Meerdink Company, Ltd.
1555 South Park Avenue
Neenah, WI 54956
(920) 725-0955 Worldwide • (800) 635-6499 U.S. & Canada
www.horseinfo.com

Printed in the United States of America

To War Admiral,
whose great heart came to him through
the legendary Domino and Sweep and
races today through his daughters
and their descendants.

Acknowledgments

Research takes a lot of help and networking to accomplish the goal of expanding our knowledge. In the past eight years, many people and horses have contributed to what we have learned. At the top of the list must come my partner and friend, Dr. Fred Fregin, who has generously shared his wisdom, intellect, compassion and understanding with a sometimes hyper-inquisitive journalist who was chasing scientific ideas like they were clues in a murder mystery. Without his help, we would never have learned the things we have. He has kept the project on an even keel carefully gathering ECGs and bringing his 25+ years of experience in equine cardiology to bear on the hearts we have measured and the pedigrees we have researched. University of Kentucky geneticist Dr. Gus Cothran kept our research on a sound genetic basis and was a constant resource for understanding what we found in the field.

The generosity of John Harris and Harris Farms greatly increased our knowledge of the way the heart was inherited. Eclipse Champion Tiznow, foaled at Harris Farms, is a perfect example of what can happen when speed is allied with great heart. Penny Chenery, whose great horse, Secretariat, started us down this trail, has also been an amazing resource.

Amy Owens first started me down the road to understanding the influence of heart in the racing Quarter Horse. The AQHA in Amarillo, Texas, was instrumental in our work with Quarter Horses. Richard Chamberlain, editor of the American Quarter Horse Racing Journal, along with Terry Stidger and Tawanna Walker of his staff, were of invaluable assistance. Dr. Dan Lucas, with his understanding of genetics and the value the X Factor could have in breeding top racehorses, was a great resource as we measured the family links of his horses. Bonnie and Scoop

Vessels of Vessels Stallion Farm were of considerable help in learning what great heart meant in a Quarter Horse.

I received research help from many people including: Sandy Clark, Keri Basham, Phil Bourke, Susan Larkin, Mike Becker, Barry Keown, Anne Peters, Margaret Neal, and William and Kristie Jakeman and their wonderful broodmare, Bonnie's Poker, who gave War Admiral's heart to Silver Charm. Others contributing include Glori Ekker, Sue Brown, and Leonie Ommundson, whose research with high-speed treadmills and its impact on cardiovascular conditioning was invaluable.

I want to thank James and Kellye Pikul for the use of their farm, Tierra Bonita, where Man 'o Sheba was foaled.

The Kentucky Horse Park was generous in letting us measure the hearts of some of racing's greatest champions.

When it came to understanding the role heart played in trotters, many Kentucky farms and breeders, including Hunterton Farm and Castleton Farm, were open in sharing what they had seen and experienced in breeding outstanding trotters.

A special thanks must go to Phyllis Rogers and Cathy Schenck of Keeneland Library, whose efforts to find a temporary shelter for the amazing Keeneland Library collection while a new library is being built was a godsend not only to myself, but to all other turf writers and researchers.

I also wish to acknowledge the generosity of the Thoroughbred Times in letting us use pictures from their vast collection of historic Thoroughbred photos. It was greatly appreciated. Laura Tucker, their librarian, was especially helpful.

And last, but by no means least, I have to thank my son, Kelly Borkert, and his wife, Tina, for their unstinting support and for housing my life in their new home while I gallivant all over the country.

CONTENTS

"Round hoofed, short joined, fetlocks shag and long.
Broad breast, full eye, small head and nostril wide
High crest, short ears, straight legs and passing strong
Thin mane, thick tail, broad buttocks, tender hide.
Look, what a horse should have he did not lack
Save a proud rider on so proud a back."

Author unknown

Chapter 1

The X Factor

Throughout the centuries, champion racehorses have been described as having "great heart." Thanks to recent genetic discoveries, we now know that this was more than just a term for determination and courage . . . that indefinable something that keeps certain horses going when others have fallen back.

There has never been, and perhaps never will be, a definitive answer to the question of what makes a champion. There are too many variables and too many ways to combine them. It is possible to say, however, that certain attributes seem to show up with regularity in the great champions. One such attribute is clearly a large heart.

With the death of Secretariat, arguably the greatest racehorse ever, a discovery was made at autopsy of a truly great heart, the largest ever seen. The heart was carefully examined both with the naked eye and microscopically, and found to be in perfect condition with no abnormalities except for its great size. It was just a huge engine, estimated at 22 pounds, that powered the horse often described as "moving like a tremendous machine."

Today, thanks to the truly great heart uncovered at the autopsy of Secretariat, it is known that "great heart" really is a physical description of an extraordinary heart found in certain Thoroughbreds, Quarter Horses, Standardbreds, Arabians, and Morgans. This heart has passed down the female line on the X chromosome from the legendary Eclipse, foaled in England in 1764.

Following the tradition of burying just the head, heart and hooves of great racehorses, Eclipse was cut open by a London surgeon after his death in 1789. The heart found inside Eclipse was so much larger than those of other horses that it was weighed. Eclipse's great heart weighed 14 pounds, more than twice the normal six-pound weight of hearts of horses of that era.

Today, the normal weight of a horse's heart is 8.5 pounds. Even though Secretariat's heart was not weighed at autopsy, Dr. Thomas Swerczek, head pathologist at the University of Kentucky, estimated it at 22 pounds after finding the second-largest heart in Sham (Secretariat's Triple Crown rival) and weighing it at 18 pounds.

"I have done thousands of autopsies, and I had noticed differences in heart size in horses before we did Secretariat," said Swerczek. "I had picked up the difference in the male and female hearts and noticed that some were bigger than others. But I didn't pay much attention until Secretariat came along. He was completely out of everybody else's league. Looking back at what he had done, it was easy to put a connection to it. The heart was what made him able to do what he did. It explained how he was able to do what he did in the Belmont Stakes — a mile and a half race (Secretariat won by 31 lengths in track-record time). You would have to have a large heart to do what he did. It would be impossible for a horse with a small heart to do that."

Recalling the moment Secretariat's heart was uncovered, Swerczek said, "We just stood there in stunned silence. We couldn't believe it. The heart was perfect. There were no problems with it. It was just this huge engine."

For more than 40 years, Australian researchers have studied hearts found in racehorses and have demonstrated a strong pattern of performance correlated with large hearts. Much of the interest in heart size in Australia stemmed from the 1932 discovery of the 14-pound heart carried by the legendary Phar Lap, Australia's greatest racehorse. Until Secretariat's death, Phar Lap's heart was considered the world's benchmark. So noteworthy was that great heart that it has been encased in glass in the Australian National Museum in Canberra. The large-hearted horses in Australia, including Phar Lap, follow the X chromosome to Pocahontas and

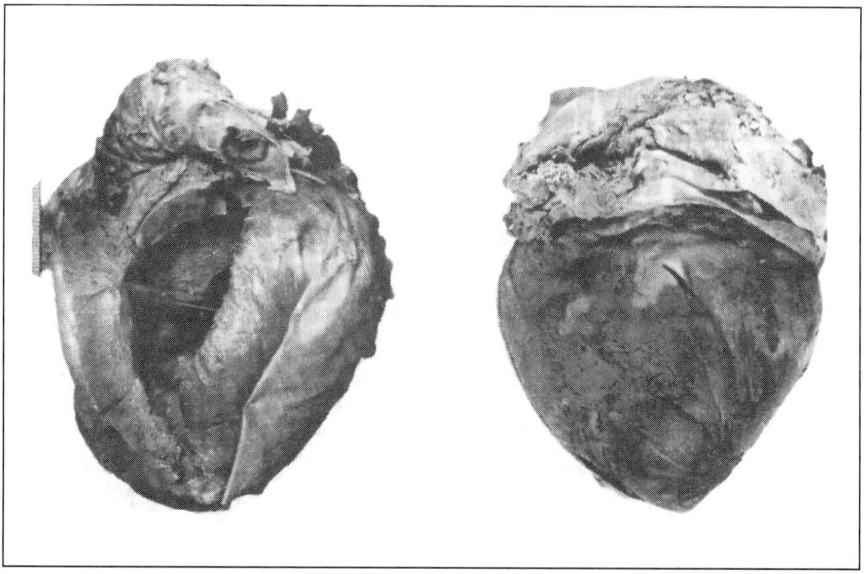

Upon his death in 1932, the heart of the legendary Phar Lap of the Australian racing circuit was found to weigh 14 pounds. On the left, the left ventricle is opened to show the 4.3 centimeters-thick walls. On the right, the pericardium has been turned up. Below, Phar Lap is shown in action.

From The Evolution of the Endurance, Speed and Staying Power of the Racehorse *by W.J. Stewart McKay, M.B., M.Ch., B.Sc. (Charles Scribner's Sons, 1933)*

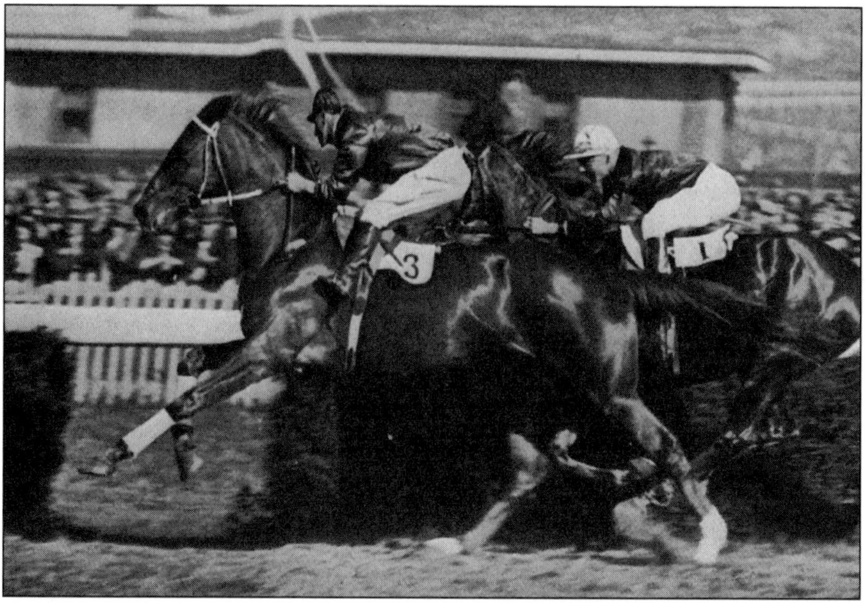

Eclipse. Phar Lap's sire Winkie went to Pocahontas through his third dam Hilarity, by Pocahontas' son King Tom. Phar Lap's heart was the same size as Eclipse's heart. A daughter of Stockwell, Lady Chester, was the dam of Chester, a great Australian racehorse and sire. Araucaria produced Apremont, who exercised considerable influence on the bloodstock of New Zealand. Sandal, dam of Instep, ancestress of Aurum, Auraria, Desert Gold, Nadean and other noted Australian horses, was a daughter of Stockwell.

On the track, Phar Lap proved triumphant so many times that his mysterious death was thought to be the result of foul play. Unfortunately, he was gelded so he never passed on his great heart.

However, when Australian researchers tried to relate their findings about large hearts to U.S. veterinarians in the 1960s, they were laughed at because they couldn't go out and pick out horses with large hearts. From their studies, they felt that large hearts represented a sex-linked characteristic, with the main influence coming from the dams, but they didn't know where that characteristic came from.

Today, the average Thoroughbred heart weighs 8.5 pounds. In an ongoing study involving myself; equine cardiologist Dr. Fred Fregin, director of the Marion du Pont Scott Equine Research Hospital in Leesburg, Virginia; and geneticist Dr. Gus Cothran of the University of Kentucky, we have measured by ECG more than 1,000 hearts.

Australian studies rank heart scores in horses according to size. Heart scores of 103 and below are considered small. Heart scores from 104-116 are considered normal. Female hearts from 117 and above are considered large. Male hearts from 120 and above are considered large. In our study, we found heart scores ranging from 100 to 160. In terms of heart weight, that translates from 5.5 pounds to 16 pounds — quite a range in heart size.

The largest heart in our study so far was found in Thoroughbred champion Key to the Mint. He carried the Princequillo heart and had a heart score of 157-160. We also measured an outstanding daughter of Key to the Mint who has produced two millionaire daughters, and she had the exact same heart size as her sire. Most of the Princequillo hearts were between 147 and 160. The other three super heartlines — those of War Admiral, Blue Larkspur and Mahmoud — were between 140-150. Hearts of 140 and above are considered very large and are generally found in very successful racehorses.

Although we don't have a heart score on Secretariat, based on his estimated heart weight at the time of autopsy his heart score would have been around 180. Even in horses carrying the stallion's heart, we have not found a heart close to that size. It might be that Secretariat, in his heart as well as in his other physical characteristics, was a genetic anomaly. But if his heart hadn't been so far out of the norm, we might never have discovered what we have about this genetic mutation that produces a high-performance heart.

After measuring more than 1,000 horses with an ECG, Dr. Fregin has found the X Factor to be 100 percent consistent, a rarity in scientific research. We have been able to track the large heart from sire to daughter to granddaughter and grandson and to great-granddaughter and great-grandson. The heart scores on certain lines have been so consistent that we were able to determine which X chromosome was expressed and to identify the four above-mentioned "super hearts" found in today's pedigrees.

Following the publication of my first article about Secretariat's heart in the spring of 1993, I began to search for the source of the great heart. Dr. Cothran said that if large hearts were a sex-linked characteristic as the Australians believed, then the characteristic could be traced to a single source and would be a genetic mutation found on the X chromosome, which passes through the female line.

After months of intense pedigree research, I found a genetic connection on the X chromosome from Secretariat's large heart to Eclipse's large heart found at his death 200 years before. Most large hearts could be traced through a mare named Pocahontas, foaled in England in 1837, and went to the same daughter of Eclipse, Everlasting, both through her sire Glencoe and on her tail-female line.

A few horses trace back to Eclipse through other Glencoe daughters and through Lexington daughters. The great sire Domino carried the large heart of Eclipse through the Glencoe mare Judith and passed it on through his daughters. In a recent discovery, Lexington was found to descend from an unnamed daughter of Eclipse foaled in 1785.

This connection was true for all large hearts found in Thoroughbreds all over the world. Because the breed was founded in England, which for centuries had widespread colonies around the world, Eclipse's great heart was shipped all over the globe through his daughters. Glencoe, who came to Kentucky after siring Pocahontas in England, spread his large heart through his daughters in America at the same time that Lexington was passing on his heart in America through his daughters.

Definitions

X and Y chromosomes, single copy and double copy:
Genetically, there are two sex-linked chromosomes in each horse. Males have an X chromosome, which they receive from their dams and pass to their daughters, and a Y chromosome, which they inherit from their sires and pass to their sons. Females have two X chromosomes.

The Y chromosome is much smaller than the X chromosome and carries a smaller amount of inheritable material. It is basically a sex determinant and when thrown into the mix at the moment of creation makes that individual a male. If the sire contributes an X chromosome, the resulting foal is a female.

Because the large-heart characteristic is on the X chromosome, large-hearted stallions can only pass on the trait to their daughters, who carry their sire's X chromosome and one of the two X chromosomes carried by their dam. Whichever X chromosome is dominant is the one that is expressed. If a mare is a single-copy mare (meaning she carries the large heart on only one of her X chromosomes), she could pass on either the large-hearted X chromosome or the small-hearted X chromosome to her sons and daughters. The ideal broodmare has the large-heart trait on both X chromosomes. If the mare is bred to a large-hearted sire, she will always produce large-hearted foals. Her daughters also will be double-copy mares.

X Factor:
Term geneticists use to describe the female X chromosome, which is attributed with creating the large hearts found in outstanding racehorses.

Heart Score:
Term coined by Australian researcher Dr. James Steel to communicate his findings of the heart size on the electrocardiogram, which was gained by a correlation of heart weight, stroke volume, cardiac output and aerobic power.

Chapter 2

The Origin of Heart Score

Before the beginning of modern genetics, horse breeding had been a matter of shrewd guesswork and traditional practices. The guesswork had more often failed to produce champions than it had succeeded. There was agreement that certain traits were heritable, but it was unclear how they were inherited.

Systematic data was needed in two areas: Was there some common bond among the large-hearted horses of modern times and the storied champions of history? If there was a bond, was it a predictable one?

Before that question could be addressed, however, the more basic question had to be answered: Was that large-heart characteristic truly a contributing factor in performance?

The collection of the data to answer that question began almost by accident. In 1953, Australian researcher Dr. James D. Steel, a professor and senior lecturer in veterinary medicine at the University of Sydney, first began using electrocardiography in studies of herbivores (grazing animals). The herbivores he was studying were located mostly in the racing stables of Maurice McCarten, an Australian racehorse trainer. As Steel's work became more widely known, it was extended to other racing trainers.

Initially, Steel was investigating whether racehorses suffered from heart disease when he noticed an unusual characteristic on the electrocardiogram (ECG) of a leading racehorse of the time, Prince Courtauld.

By using an ECG examination, Steel was able to determine that the heart size of the racehorse was greater than that of a much less successful horse, three-year-old Momote. It was during this time that he coined the term "heart score" to communicate his

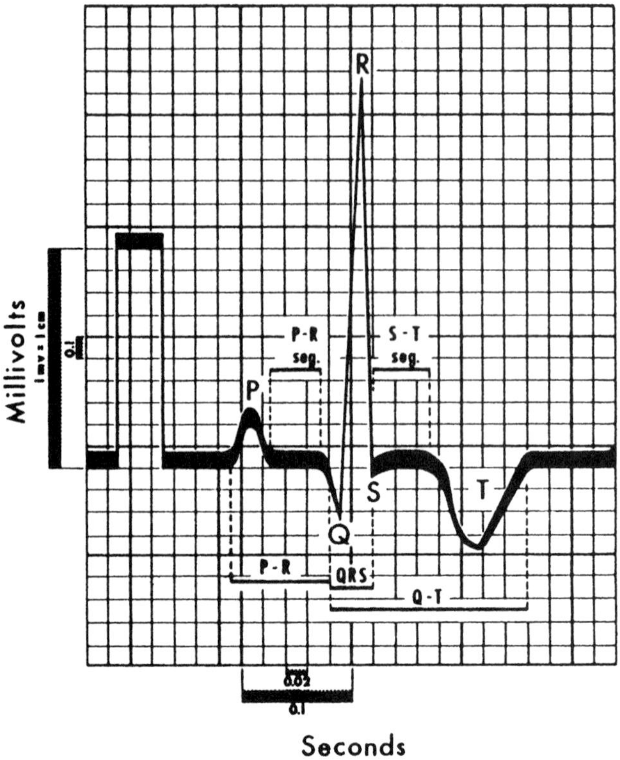

The difference between a small heart and a large heart as shown on the ECG is the width of the QRS wave. The large heart will have a wide QRS baseline. The small heart will show a much narrower baseline.

findings of the heart size on the ECG, which were gained by a correlation of heart weight, stroke volume, cardiac output, and aerobic power.

In doing the ECGs on these two horses, Steel noticed unusually wide QRS complexes in the electrocardiogram of Prince Courtauld. A comparison between this ECG and Momote's showed a heart score of 130 for Prince Courtauld and 86 for Momote.

To summarize the differences in the width of the QRS complex and to communicate his findings to people who were unfamiliar with ECG terminology, Steel used the term "heart score" to indicate the mean of the QRS duration recorded from the standard limb leads.

The QRS complex is a series of waves inscribed in the electrocardiogram when the bulk of the heart (ventricles) is electrically activated during each beat. This activation occurs naturally every time the heart beats.

The ECG is recorded on paper moving at a constant speed. A wider QRS complex represents a longer activation time. The larger the mass (weight of the heart), the longer it takes to activate it and the wider the QRS complex and the bigger the heart score.

This was the critical connection. A wider QRS complex is evidence of a large heart and that large heart can pump more blood

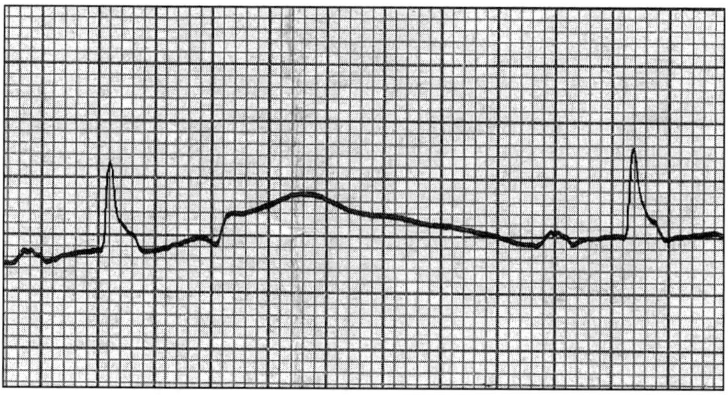

The ECG for Moscow Ballet shows a very wide QRS wave. Moscow Ballet was measured and found to have a heart score of 147.

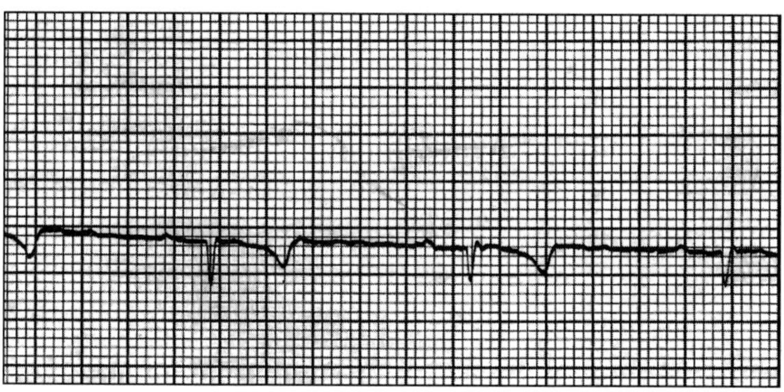

The ECG for horse with a small heart shows a narrow QRS Wave.

with each beat (stroke volume) and therefore per minute (cardiac output).

Through his findings, Steel determined that male horses with a heart score of 120 or more were in the large-heart category. Fillies and mares with a heart score of 116 or more were in the large-heart score category. Horses with heart scores of 103 or less were deemed in the small-heart category, and heart scores in between these two categories were considered medium- or normal-sized.

Steel's research, therefore, had established a way of noninvasively determining the size of a horse's heart. With this technique available, Steel began to seek a relationship between the heart score and performance. He compiled and studied the racing performance and ECGs of 306 Thoroughbreds. In a preliminary paper in 1957, some of these findings were published. The major part of his work, based on the ECGs of 2,500 Thoroughbreds, was published six years later.

Steel had established the crucial link between heart score, heart size and performance. It remained for others to explore that link. If a link existed between Sham and Secretariat, for instance, the implications would be enormous.

The project which sought to, and did, establish the link is detailed later in this book, but, in brief, it was discovered that both stallions were out of daughters of Princequillo, one of the most successful broodmare sires of the 20th century. Because Australian researchers believed the characteristic was sex-linked, or passed along the X chromosome from mother to son to daughter to son and daughter, this was significant.

In addition to leaving a legacy of racing records, Secretariat's most important contribution may well be his great heart which opened the door to the discovery of important clues to a genetic link between large hearts and the X chromosome. The exploration of that link, however, can best be understood by first exploring some of the work that preceded it.

Chapter 3

The Link Between Heart Score and Performance

In Australia, a growing number of veterinarians studied under Steel and subsequently practiced his brand of equine cardiology. From this group came increasing recognition of the value of heart score in assessing potential for strenuous exercise performance, not only in horse racing but also in human athletics, greyhound racing, equine endurance riding, and three-day eventing. For many years in New Zealand, the heart score has been incorporated into the routine cardiology of racehorses.

According to Dr. Anthony Stewart, who studied under Steel and is today one of Australia's leading experts in heart research, the high incidence of large heart scores in successful racehorses suggests that a large heart is a desirable characteristic for racing in the highest class.

In an Australian study of 18 Thoroughbreds, who among them were successful in 22 runnings of either the Victoria Racing Club Victoria Derby (Aust-G1) or the Australian Jockey Club Derby (Aust-G1), it was found that 17 had large heart scores between 120 and 136, inclusive. In a similar study of 20 winners of either the Caulfield Cup (Aust-G1) or Melbourne Cup (Aust-G1), 15 were found to have heart scores of 120 or more. These were among Australia's most prestigious races.

The heart size indicated in the heart score, Stewart said, appears to contribute approximately 23 percent of the overall quality of the racehorse. "The heart score provides one easily measured factor among many of significance in the assessment of potential for racing," he said.

Further confirmation of the relationship between the heart score and racing performance has now come from workers independently of the groups in Australia and New Zealand.

"From Denmark, Nielsen and Vibe-Petersen reported highly significant correlations between heart score and both kilometre time and stakes money won by trotting horses," said Stewart. "Guarded support has also come from Physick-Sheard and Hendren, studying Standardbreds in Canada. In the United Kingdom, Leadon, Cunningham, Mahon and Todd reported a significant correlation between heart score and Timeform ratings in 71 three-year-olds, but not in 70 two-year-olds, yet, strangely, both correlation coefficients (r-0.359 and 0.320 respectively) statistically seemed to be highly significant."

Stewart said not all groups have been successful in detecting a relationship between heart score and racing performance. He cited a study done in the United States by Gross, Muir, Pipers, and Hamlin which recognized no correlation. He pointed out, however, that the study comprised only 12 Thoroughbreds whose heart scores had been obtained when they were yearlings. Since a horse's heart grows until he is four years old, Stewart said, anyone attempting to use the measurement of a yearling's heart is merely guessing at what the size might eventually be.

In addition to Thoroughbreds, Australian researchers and other groups abroad have studied Standardbreds and documented the same relationship between large hearts and high heart scores to performance that was found in the Thoroughbreds.

A group of researchers in Australia did a study on families of Standardbreds in the 1960s. Stewart said the researchers determined from what they discovered with measurements of the horses that the large-heart characteristic appeared to be a sex-linked co-dominant genetic trait on the X chromosome. They found the heart size of the female offspring was either from the sire or the dam or a blending of the two with the colt's heart size coming from the dam. The large-heart characteristic is felt to be just as valuable in a trotting horse as in a flat-racing animal. In the study of 195 trotting horses by Nielsen and Vibe-Petersen in Denmark, they reported a mean correlation coefficient between kilometer time and heart score of 0.47. Using the correlation between the heart score and the performance parameter, highest standard of race won by the horse, the figure indicates that 22 percent of the performance parameter can be attributed to the heart score.

These estimates put the heart score theory in reasonable context against other factors contributing to the performance and quality of the racehorse.

"The estimates of 22-23 percent still leave approximately 77 percent of the quality to be derived from other factors, as many of which as possible should be taken into account when assessing the animal," said Stewart. "Yet amongst all these variables, for one easily-measured factor — the heart score — to account for 23 percent provides a useful contribution to the overall assessment of potential for racing."

In the British study done by Leadon, Cunningham, Mahon, and Todd, Stewart said it was noted that horses grouped according to heart score showed an increasing minimum Timeform rating with each increment in heart score; e.g., as the heart score rose, a higher minimum performance was achieved within the group of horses with that heart score.

"In an individual horse with a high heart score there is a danger that this may engender unrealistically high expectations unless one takes into account the many other factors contributing to the quality and performance of the racehorse," said Stewart. "Of more practical use may be the fact that horses with lower heart scores do not perform as well or consistently in high-class racing as do horses with high heart scores, and a guarded prognosis should be made when the heart score is medium-low."

The incidence of large heart scores is approximately 25 percent in the overall racehorse population, Stewart said.

"If a high heart score is an important characteristic for performance, its incidence among successful horses should be substantially higher," he said, adding that this effect has been shown to be present in several studies, including those done with the Victoria Derby, AJC Derby, Melbourne Cup, and Caulfield Cup.

"In studying elite trotters competing in the 1979 International race, the Copenhagen Cup, Nielsen and Vibe-Petersen found large heart scores of 124 or higher in all eight runners," said Stewart. "This incidence of 100-percent large heart scores contrasted with an incidence of 28 percent (heart score of 117 or higher) among 175 mares and stallions in the general population studied by these workers, and their mean heart score for mature mares and stallions of 110.4, with a standard deviation of 12.8.In Standardbreds, Steel too had noted the occurrence of consistently high heart scores in the horses contesting the 1960 Yonkers International Pacing Series in New York, and also in better-performed pacers here at Harold Park."

In Australia, a retrospective study of Thoroughbreds was conducted. The weight-for-age races during the Spring Racing Carnival in Melbourne were taken to be representative of Australian racing of the highest class. In this study, 35 weight-for-age winners with recorded heart scores were identified and 31 had heart scores between 120 and 140, inclusive. The other four had heart scores of 113. "Thus 89 percent of this population of high-class winners had large heart scores," said Stewart.

From these statistics, he said, again it may be concluded that large heart scores are a desirable characteristic for racing in the highest class. But, he cautioned, never forget the horse with the normal-sized heart, that is so superbly endowed with other characteristics as to overcome any advantage lost from a smaller heart.

"From the statistics, however, in an industry so oriented toward odds, one may conclude that in high-class racing the chances of success for a horse with a low heart score are correspondingly lower," he said.

Famous Racehorses' Heart Weights & Scores

Name of Horse	Heart Score	Heart Weight	
Eclipse (ch.h. 1764)	14 lbs		
Phar Lap (ch.g. 1926	14 lbs		
Secretariat (ch.h. 1970)	22 lbs		
Sham (ch.h. 1970)	18 lbs*		
Star Kingdom (ch.h. 1946)	14 lbs		
Mill Reef (b.h. 1968)	16.94 lbs*		
Easy Goer (ch.h. 1986)	15 lbs		
Althea (ch.m. 1981)	15 lbs		
Hyperion (ch.h. 1930)		133	
Moscow Ballet (b.h. 1982)			147
Soviet Problem (ch.m. 1990)		150	
The Last Red (ch.m. 1993-twin)		140	
Desert Secret (IRE)(b.h. 1969)		140	
Key To The Mint (b.h. 1969)	15.8 lbs	160	
Northern Dancer (b.h. 1961)		150	
Killaloe (b.m. 1970)	12.9 lbs		
Tulloch (AUS)(b.h. 1954)	13.5 lbs	136	
Manikato (AUS)(ch.g. 1975)		123	
Kingston Town (AUS)(bk.g. 1976)		130	

** Some pathological enlargement. Such enlargement can add two to three pounds or more to the heart weight.*

According to a study conducted by Australian scientists comparing heart score to heart weight at autopsy, the following table was established:

Comparing Heart Score and Heart Weight

Heart Score	Heart Weight
100	6.6 lbs
110	7.36 lbs
120	10.12 lbs
130	11.88 lbs
140	13.64 lbs
150	15.4 lbs
160	17.16 lbs

Chapter 4

The 120 Heart Score Advantage

To be useful to horse breeders, heart size must be quantified. Steel and Stewart have both reported results from studies demonstrating a relationship between high heart score and heart weight. Heart scores of individual horses were found to vary from 86 to 146, with heart weights from 1.9 kg (4.18 pounds) to 6.1 kg (13.42 pounds), with a highly significant correlation between heart score and heart weight.

In 1963, Steel reported a strong correlation between the QRS duration and the heart weight at autopsy in 34 racehorses ($r_{32} = + 0.89$, $P < 0.001$). By 1970 the number of autopsies studied in the relationship between heart score and heart weight had increased to 55, with a slight increase in the correlation coefficient ($r_{53} = 0.92$, $P < 0.001$). From these studies, they were able to establish a table of averages relating heart score to heart weight. In this table, a heart score of 100 is equal to a weight of 3.0 kg. One kg is equal to 2.2 pounds, so a 100 heart score would relate to a 6.6 pound heart. A heart score of 110 is 3.8 kg (7.36 pounds), 120 is 4.6 kg (10.12 pounds), 130 is 5.4 kg (11.88 pounds), 140 is 6.2 kg (13.64 pounds), 150 is 7 kg (15.4 pounds) and 160 is 7.8 kg (17.16 pounds).

When he died, Mill Reef was found to have a heart that weighed 7.7 kg (16.94 pounds). Based on the Australian scale, that would give him a heart score of approximately 158. Based on this scale, Secretariat's heart score could be estimated at 180. Sham's heart weighed 18 pounds at autopsy but it had some pathological enlargement, so it would probably be in the 150 range.

In the Australian table, the mean heart score was 111.5 plus or minus 1.45 milliseconds (msec; points in a heart score). The mean heart weight was 3.92 kg (8.6 pounds) plus or minus 0.104 kg (.23 pounds). From these studies it was concluded that individual heart scores of 120 or more represent hearts that are larger than average and heart scores of 103 or less represent hearts smaller than average. Stewart said these averages may be modified slightly to take sex difference into account. The mean heart scores of fillies and mares are approximately four msec less than those of male horses. Thus in fillies and mares, a heart score of 116 or more represents large hearts.

The relationships between heart scores and heart weight in the racehorse support the conclusion drawn by Wilson and Herman in 1930 that the "QRS interval is an accurate measure of the time required for the ventricular muscle to pass into the active state." As a result, it can be concluded that a longer QRS duration indicates a larger mass of ventricular muscle.

This has been demonstrated in other species as well. The significant relationships of the heart score to cardiac transverse diameter in Olympic athletes and to heart weight in greyhounds have confirmed the value of heart score as an indicator of heart size. Studies correlating the heart score and aerobic power of high-class athletes further suggested a relationship between these two estimates, Stewart said, perhaps through a common relationship to cardiac output.

Shortly before his death, Steel visited the Japan Racing Association Equine Health Laboratory where he undertook some preliminary studies regarding cardiac output and heart score in horses. According to Stewart, these early observations led Steel to estimate a relationship between stroke volume, heart weight, and heart score in the horses he studied, which led to the table relating heart score to heart weight. In addition to those two factors, Steel also measured the stroke volume and cardiac output of horses at maximum exercise, assuming a heart rate of 200 beats per minute.

The difference in heart score between 100 and 120 may be reflecting much greater differences in cardiac function in terms of stroke volume and cardiac output than might have been expected from an apparent difference in heart score of 20 percent.

Hence, in a functional sense, Stewart said, "One should expect very different exercise performance from the horse with the large heart, with an estimated stroke volume of a liter or more, compared with the horse with a small heart, estimated to pump only half a liter or so."

To keep the information gleaned in terms of heart score and racing performance in perspective of the galloping horse, one must consider the metabolic demands of the skeletal muscles. Unlike the human athlete, the racehorse has skeletal muscle fibers with high oxidative metabolism for both sprinting and staying.

"Thus a high cardiac output during exercise represents an enormous advantage to the racehorse with the large heart, whether it be for speed or stamina," said Stewart. "It may now be concluded that the relationship between heart score and stroke volume, the high heart rate during racing, and the large oxygen requirements of the horse galloping provide a sound physiological basis for the relationships between the heart score and racing performance in all distances over which the Thoroughbred races."

The large heart has been a consistent characteristic found in the very top racehorses. "That is one of the reasons we are conducting this study," said equine cardiologist Dr. Fregin. "You don't usually find small hearts in the best runners. We've measured more than 1,000 horses now and the evidence has been very consistent. Dr. Steel and Dr. Stewart have shown significant correlation between heart score and racing performance in their research that indicated that a large heart was at least one factor that could be associated with a successful racehorse. We started on this trail more than 40 years ago. Now maybe we can finally put it all together and see where it starts. We have long been selecting horses and breeding horses because of their racing performance and what we may have actually been doing has been to unknowingly select and breed animals with large hearts."

There have been notable exceptions like Bold Ruler and Caro, who were found to have normal-sized hearts at autopsy. There will always be individuals that have such superb characteristics in other areas as to make up for smaller hearts.

Chapter 5

How to Measure Hearts

To find out what is inside a prospective athlete or breeding animal, you have to look. Science has given us ways to check the bones, joints, hearts and lungs of potential athletes. Whether an ultrasound or electrocardiogram is used, if you want to breed an outstanding performance athlete or purchase a potential racehorse you need to get all available data about the engine that powers that horse. A good, healthy heart in a racehorse is like having a high-powered V-8 engine in your car. You will never get left at the red light with a 351 Cleveland four-bolt Main engine under your hood. A large heart in a racehorse means he will have a higher cardiac output, which means he will still have plenty of gas at the finish line.

Heart measurements have become important in major sales of yearlings and two-year-olds. It is evident at the best sales like Keeneland's July and September yearling sales, Saratoga's sale in August, and two-year-old sales from coast to coast. Kentucky Derby winner Silver Charm was measured as a yearling before being purchased, as was Horse of the Year Favorite Trick. Both have extraordinary hearts.

The most common way of measuring horses' hearts at the sales is by using an ultrasound machine in a manner developed by radiologist Norman Rantanen. Because the heart increases in size until the horse is four years old, the measurement of yearlings at the top sales is done with a mathematical formula to predict the final outcome. But when a yearling already has a large heart, the buyer knows he has a good one.

While it is always best to select a mare with a good performance record for breeding, this isn't always necessary. There are always individuals that for some reason —- injury, finances or whatever —- didn't have outstanding performance records but still have outstanding pedigrees with the right heartlines.

An example is the mare Ride the Trails by Prince John, who traces to Blue Larkspur through her paternal great-granddam Banish Fear and to Princequillo through her broodmare sire Sir Gaylord's dam, Somethingroyal, and to War Admiral through her tail-female line to her great-grandam Portage, a daughter of War Admiral.

Ride the Trails never raced but she produced the champion Cozzene as well as black-type winning daughters Mochila, Movin' Money and Ivy Road and winner Mesabi, all of whom have gone on to produce black-type winners.

Turf history is full of mares that either were never raced or were unsuccessful at racing, but still went on to produce winners. Playmate, who only placed at four, still produced the Irish champion two-year-old Woodman, who has gone on to be a

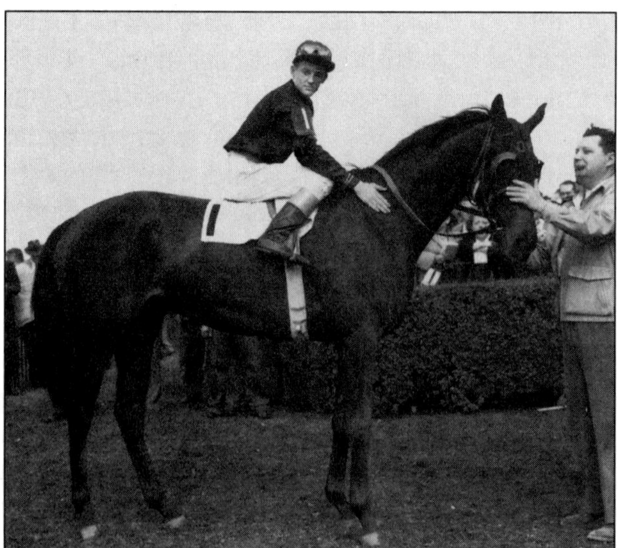

Photo courtesy of the Keeneland Library

Busanda (War Admiral x Businesslike) the double-copy dam of Buckpasser successful sire. Playmate carried the large-hearted X chromosome from her sire, Buckpasser out of Busanda, by War Admiral out of Businesslike, by Blue Larkspur. Buckpasser is one of the very best proponents of the large heart through his double-copy dam. Using the ECG and autopsy reports, large hearts were found consistently in the maternal grandsons of Buckpasser.

While the gene-tracing project conducted by Fregin, Cothran and myself has found larger heart scores than the Australians, it also has had access to the very best bloodstock in the world. The horses with the very highest heart scores all trace back to the four largest heart lines and were, unless stopped by injury, all top performers, including a number of champions.

Among the more than 1,000 horses measured in the project, the heart score ranges were 100 to 157 for mares, 117-160 for stallions, and 117-143 for two-year-olds in training.

One yearling was measured at 14 months with a heart score of 130, and an eight-month-old Quarter Horse filly was measured and found to have a heart score of 120, indicating a potential for very large hearts at maturity. We measured two two-year-old fillies in California and found two extraordinary hearts. One, Trifecta Box, a daughter of Boone's Mill, had a heart score of 140, which could mature to 150-160. We believe this is Secretariat's heart, as we were able to measure her dam and that was the only line in her pedigree capable of passing on that great heart. Another filly, Political Favor, had an even larger heart with a heart score of 143, which could conceivably reach 160. Because we had the heart score of her sire and dam, the most likely source of that great heart was Domino through her broodmare sire Stalwart. Stalwart's name has a certain irony if he is passing that great heart. Tale of Two Hearts, a daughter of Desert Secret out of the tiny twin The Last Red, recorded a heart score of 147 when measured at three years. This is the My Charmer heart passed by Seattle Slew.

The smallest heart scores were found either in failed racehorses or in mares carrying a single copy. Two mares that were measured and found to have small- to normal-sized hearts had one X chromosome line with good heart lines and had produced large-hearted offspring. With single-copy mares, it simply depends on which X comes up as dominant in the genetic spin of the wheel.

In choosing an ECG to measure a horse's heart size, the heart score categories are as follows: 103 and below is considered small; 104 to 117 is considered normal-sized; and in fillies 116 and up is considered large, while colts are considered to have large hearts with heart scores from 120 and up.

"Electrocardiography, which once was the exclusive tool of the cardiologist, is a relatively inexpensive and noninvasive tool which can be used by the veterinary practitioner and his staff," said

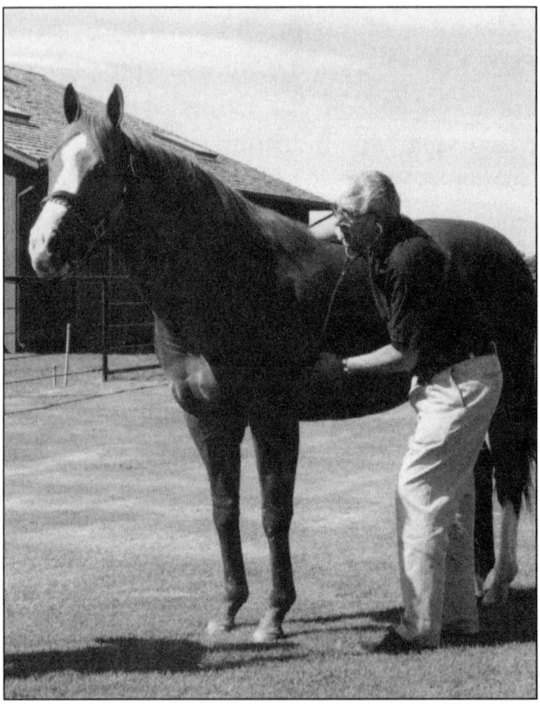

Dr. Fred Fregin, Director of the Marion duPont Scott Equine Medical Center, examines Rare Form.

Photo by Amy Owens

Dr. Fregin, who conducted all of the gene project measurements on the ECG.

"The form of the equine ECG will be altered significantly by variations in the activity of the autonomic nervous system (excitement, for example) and by changes in forelimb positioning. It is important that the horse be examined in quiet, familiar surroundings, with the forelimbs kept parallel to each other and perpendicular to the long axis of the body."

In the study, most of the measurements were done in each horse's own stall, but some mares' were done in paddocks near their pasture. The most important thing was to keep them quiet in order to obtain a good tracing on the ECG. Nervous head-tossing or jerks or twitches could distort the tracing.

The author was involved in the study and my job was to be at the horse's head and keep him or her calm while Fregin listened for heart sounds then set the ECG leads and ran the tape.

I must have a smell that horses relate to because they all liked to rest their noses on my chest, mares and stallions alike. When we were doing 53 horses in California in just a few days, by the end of the day the small of my back was killing me and the horse manager was worrying that my sweatshirt would act as a vector if any of the horses had germs.

But it worked. Even Key to the Mint, who hadn't been in for a year and came in rearing, reacted positively to my smell and my voice with his eyes visibly softening and his lids drooping as he rested his nose on my chest. Gainesway's veterinarian, Norman Umphenour, said I was "mesmerizing" the stallion.

While Key to the Mint was my most dramatic conquest, I have found in the past three years that horses of any age or sex are quite attracted to vanilla perfume. After a visit to Saratoga, where I discovered that wonder of crème brulee, I found a large bottle of perfume by the same name which was very enthusiastically received by all breeds and ages of horses. I think that perfume might work almost as well as any horse whisperer.

In describing the technique he uses with the ECG, Fregin said, "Patient cables with a total length of 20 to 25 feet are used to allow the ECG equipment to be placed in a remote location outside of the box stall. The limb and chest leads should be five feet in length and accommodate larger horses. Alligator clips fixed to the ECG leads may be attached directly to the skin after vigorous application of an electrode paste of gel. Discomfort to the horse will be minimized by smoothing (rounding off) the serrated edges

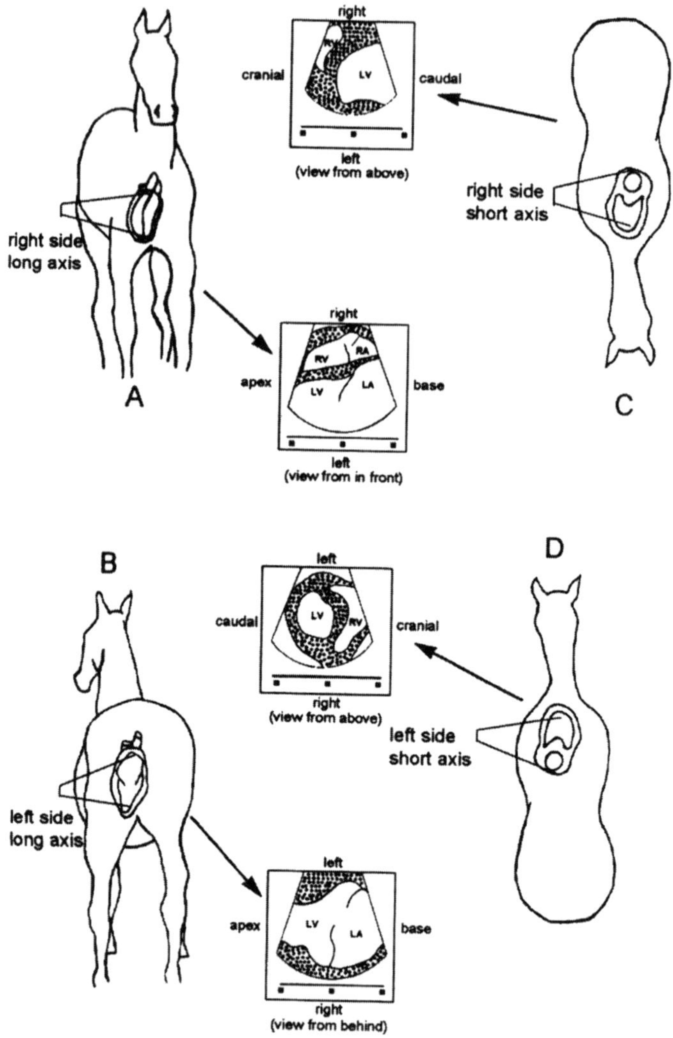

A) Schematic illustration of imaging and projection of long axis planes recorded from the right side of the chest. The scan is viewed from in front of the horse. RA: right atrium; RV: right ventricle; LA: left atrium; LV: left ventricle. B) Schematic illustration of imaging and projection of long axis planes recorded from the left side of the chest. The scan is viewed from behind the horse. LA: left atrium; LV: left ventricle. C) Schematic illustration of imaging and projections of short axis planes recorded from the right side of the chest. The scan is viewed from above the horse. RV: right ventricle; LV: left ventricle: D) Schematic illustration of imaging and projections of short axis planes recorded from the left side of the chest. The scan is viewed from above the horse. RV: right ventricle; LV: left ventricle.

of the alligator clips, by insuring that the maximum amount of skin is grasped, and by reducing tension or movement of the leads. The electrodes are placed on the caudal aspect of the forelimb approximately 15 cm below the level of the olecranon and on the hind limbs, distal or lateral to the stifle joint. The standard bipolar limb leads recorded are right foreleg and left foreleg (lead I), right foreleg and left hind leg (lead II), and left foreleg and left hind leg (lead III).

"The configuration of the wave forms in different leads depends on the direction and relative magnitude of the variations in the electrical forces generated during the cardiac cycle. These forces are determined primarily by the specialized conduction tissue (Purkinje fibers) and its influence on the spread of excitation through the myocardium. The wave forms are also influenced by the anatomic location and configuration of the heart, by the shape of the thorax, and by the electrical conductivity of the tissues between the heart and recording electrodes."

Norm Rantanen, one of the nation's top radiologists who developed the use of two-dimensional echocardiography (ultrasound) to measure the heart size of horses, has done comparison studies of the two methods, ECG and ultrasound, and found them consistent in their findings on heart size. Rantanen started measuring hearts in the Lexington, Ky., area in 1983.

"We tried the technique that the Aussies use — the ECG which is what Fred (Fregin) is using," said Rantanen. "We also tried the ultrasound and they picked the top horses in any group that we did. (Dr.) Doug Byars did the ECGs. (Byars is director of the Internal Medicine Hospital of Hagyard-Davidson-McGee Equine Medicine and Surgery in Lexington, Kentucky.) We did it on North Ridge yearlings. We went to Ireland and did a whole series of yearlings over there. Doug did the ECG and I did the ultrasound. He ranked his according to what he found and I ranked mine according to what I found. We always picked the top horses. The findings were very consistent."

When Rantanen first came to Lexington, he worked for two medical ultrasonographers who had hired him to come develop the animal ultrasound. "At that time, everybody was looking into exercise physiology and performance testing. It was the latest thing. We tried to promote that particular service and called in work daily from Washington state and a few other people and offered that to the owners and trainers and people in town as a way they could test their animals and learn something about their physiology. One of the things we were offering was cardiac tests," said Rantanen.

"That's how I got started. That is when (veterinarian David) Lambert came to me. He asked me about the procedures I was doing and I told him. That's when he asked me if I would be interested in looking at some stock. We looked primarily at two-year-olds in training. I measured horses at Don and Linda Johnson's Crescent Farm. I scanned Night Shift, now standing in Europe. He was an unraced son of Northern Dancer and had a very large heart. He had surgery on his soft palate as a yearling that was screwed up and it ruined him for racing, he said."

In developing his technique, Rantanen had the help of Dr. Anthony DeMaria, then the chief of cardiology at the University of Kentucky. "We hauled tapes to UK and Norton's Children's Hospital in Louisville where they allowed us to use their measuring devices. With their help, I came up with a technique that was reproducible in the same horse at different times and also between horses because I knew exactly where to go inside the heart."

Rantanen has measured nearly 4,000 horses since developing the use of ultrasound. "The best ones have the bigger hearts. That's what I've found over the years."

Rantanen was not surprised at the consistency of heart size found in hearts on certain lines in our project. "I knew that because of the information the Australians had published," he said. "And I believe that the broodmare has a lot to do with it. I knew there was something there, but I just didn't have the wherewithal to follow it up. I didn't have the opportunity to follow a lot of family lines. I didn't have the budget to do that.

"We did a lot at North Ridge Farm for Franklin Groves. We went there and did his yearling crops. We ranked them from top to bottom. We were hoping that he would use that to dictate which horses that he sold, but he didn't do that. A lot of horses ended up being sold to people that were right at the top of the list we made. When horses have very large hearts, you can see them as yearlings. Yearlings are identifiable."

Rantanen said when he started looking at horses' hearts, it was primarily for people who were looking for horses to race. "We looked at two-year-olds in training," he said. "After that, we started looking at younger horses. I also looked at some broodmares for Robert Sangster. But it was really hard to get people to fund it." He worked for many months without funding, just to get the technique down.

Today, Rantanen credits Lambert with having the best technique for measuring hearts. "He took the technique I developed and was able to get the financial backing to do the statistical work on it," he said. "So he knows the most. But he is doing it as a private venture and he is certainly not going to divulge his techniques."

In a report validating the use of two-dimensional echocardiography of the horse as used by Rantanen, K. Voros, J.R. Holmes, and Christine Gibbs from the University of Bristol in England wrote in the Equine Veterinary Journal that during ultrasound examinations the transducer is placed between the ribs either on the right or left side of the chest where bone and overlying lung interference can be avoided.

"The 4th and 5th intercostal spaces are referred to as caudal and the 3rd as cranial transducer locations," the report said. "In the latter position it is helpful to draw the relevant foreleg forward.

"To permit production of repeatable images of the same tomographic planes, intracardiac reference points were established. Current nomenclature in two-dimensional echocardiographic examinations refers to a long axis and a short axis view. These are really longitudinal and transverse planes respectively. The right and left long axis view were obtained with the scan plane orientated parallel to the longitudinal cardiac axis, and the short axis views were achieved by directing the beam plane perpendicular to the longitudinal cardiac axis.

"By moving the transducer from the apex to the base,

several distinct short axis levels of the heart can be imaged and are classified according to relevant anatomical landmarks. From below upwards, they are referred to as papillary muscle, chordae tendineae, mitral valve, and aortic levels respectively. In all views caudo-medial or cranio-medial angulation of the beam plane may be necessary to examine the whole range of cardiac structure.

"Regardless of which side of the chest the transducer was placed, the images were displayed on the video screen with the apex of the heart always to the left and the base (atria, great vessels) to the right. Because of this orientation, long axis images taken from the right side of the chest were projected as through the encountered tomographic planes were viewed from the cranial to the caudal part of the heart and images obtained from the left side were viewed from the caudal to the cranial part of the heart.

"Short axis images recorded from either the right or the left side of the chest were projected as though the encountered tomographic planes were viewed from above, namely from the base to the apex of the heart. Thus, short axis images obtained from the right side of the chest were displayed on the video screen with cranial echoes to the left and with cranial echoes to the right side of the screen and those taken from the left side with cranial echoes to the right and caudal echoes to the left of the screen."

The study demonstrated that two-dimensional echo-cardiography (ultrasound) was an accurate anatomical evaluation of the equine heart.

The use of the ultrasound is one more way of measuring a potential athlete's heart. Gaining that valuable information, coupled with a pedigree predicting good heartline heritability, can add that much more of an edge for success in the very expensive and competitive world of racing.

Chapter 6

The X Path

The X Factor, as the path of the large-heart genetic mutation found on the X chromosome has become known, tracks the trail of Secretariat's great heart on the X line back 200 years to another legendary sire with a phenomenal heart, Eclipse.

When a London surgeon cut Eclipse open upon his death in 1789 and found his extraordinary heart, it was a momentous occasion that made the discovery of the X Factor possible 204 years later.

Without a source to trace the heart found in Secretariat it would have remained a mystery, with an occasional extraordinary horse coming along that was described as a "freak" and could seem to perform amazing feats on the racetrack. Now, with the knowledge that there is indeed a high-performance heart present in some individuals and not in others, it is possible to breed for that specific "great heart" and increase a breeder's odds of hitting the jackpot and producing a Kentucky Derby winner.

The X Factor casts doubt on the centuries-old belief that the strength of the stallion determines the athletic potential in racehorses. Because the large-heart characteristic is on the X chromosome and males carry only one X, received from their dams, large-hearted stallions can only pass on the large-heart X chromosome to their daughters, not to their sons which receive the Y chromosome from their sires. Daughters of these stallions carry their sire's X and one of the two X chromosomes carried by their dam.

Whichever X is dominant is the one that is expressed. If a mare is a single copy (carries the large heart on only one of her X chromosomes), she could pass on either the large-heart X chromosome or the small-heart X chromosome. Depending upon which X is dominant, that mare might express either a large heart or a small heart.

This information can help breeders ensure that they take full advantage of the X Factor. Because the large-heart characteristic passes via the female line and for centuries the racing industry has judged a sire by his sons, large-hearted stallions that accomplished amazing feats on the track often have been panned when they were unable to duplicate themselves in their sons. Extraordinary Thoroughbreds such as Secretariat, Omaha, Citation and Whirlaway are examples.

Man 'o War was an exception because he was lucky enough to be bred to a mare that had a larger heart than he did. That mare, Brushup (TB), was by Sweep, who also gave his high-performance heart to Dustwhirl, dam of Whirlaway.

Sweep got his large heart from the storied stallion Domino. When conformation pictures of War Admiral, Sweep and Domino are compared, the similarity is amazing. They are all approximately the same size. War Admiral is 15.2 1/2 hands and Sweep and Domino appear to be of similar size. When you consider how few individuals Domino sired, it is miraculous how successful his great heart is in today's pedigrees and champions.

Brushup produced Man 'o War's greatest son, Triple Crown winner War Admiral. The War Admiral line has become one of the four largest heart lines in today's pedigrees (joining the Thoroughbreds Princequillo, Blue Larkspur and Mahmoud). War Admiral's heart is in Seattle Slew, broodmare sire of champion Cigar, and also fuels 1997 Kentucky Derby winner Silver Charm.

Large-hearted sires that were successful racehorses have a consistent pattern of producing better daughters than sons — and thus not being appreciated until 10 to 15 years later, when their daughters begin to produce outstanding racehorses and the stallions are recognized as prolific broodmare sires. If lucky enough to be bred to good mares with large hearts, these stallions then earn the designation of being a sire of sires — ironically taking the credit for what the mare brought into the mix.

So the key to making a sire of sires out of a successful large-hearted stallion is to mate him with mares of equal heart size. The resulting colt should have an exceptional cardiovascular system.

This is what has been done with successful Thoroughbred sire Storm Cat. A speed sire, Storm Cat is mated to large-hearted mares and gets sons that can go the classic distance. The secret to achieving status as a sire is to get the best mares. The reason the genetic mutation that produces a large heart has made its way down more than 200 years through three different breeds is because of the pattern of breeding the best to the best. Because of the pattern of performance allied to the large heart, breeders have unconsciously been breeding the large heart into their respective breeds.

When selecting mares to be bred to large-hearted sires it is important that breeders remember the tail-female line. The X chromosome the dam sends to her foal doesn't just come from the broodmare sire — it also can come from the bottom of the dam's pedigree. Because there is no way of telling which X will be sent in the genetic spin of the wheel, it is important to cover all genetic bases.

Even with pedigree experts and careful selection of breeding stock, luck still plays a big part in who breeds a champion. There are genetic black holes in many pedigrees that simply can't be planned against. This is why a double-copy mare is so valuable.

The discovery also explained what happened to history's champions when they performed wondrously on the track but were deemed failures at stud. Because the large heart is carried on the X chromosome, horses like Secretariat, Citation, Omaha and Whirlaway were only able to pass it on to their daughters and not to their sons. The industry judges a sire by his sons. Ironically, what makes that son great comes not from his sire but from his dam. But the sire gets the credit.

Great-hearted sires are often not appreciated until 10 to 15 years after they've gone to stud and their daughters start producing

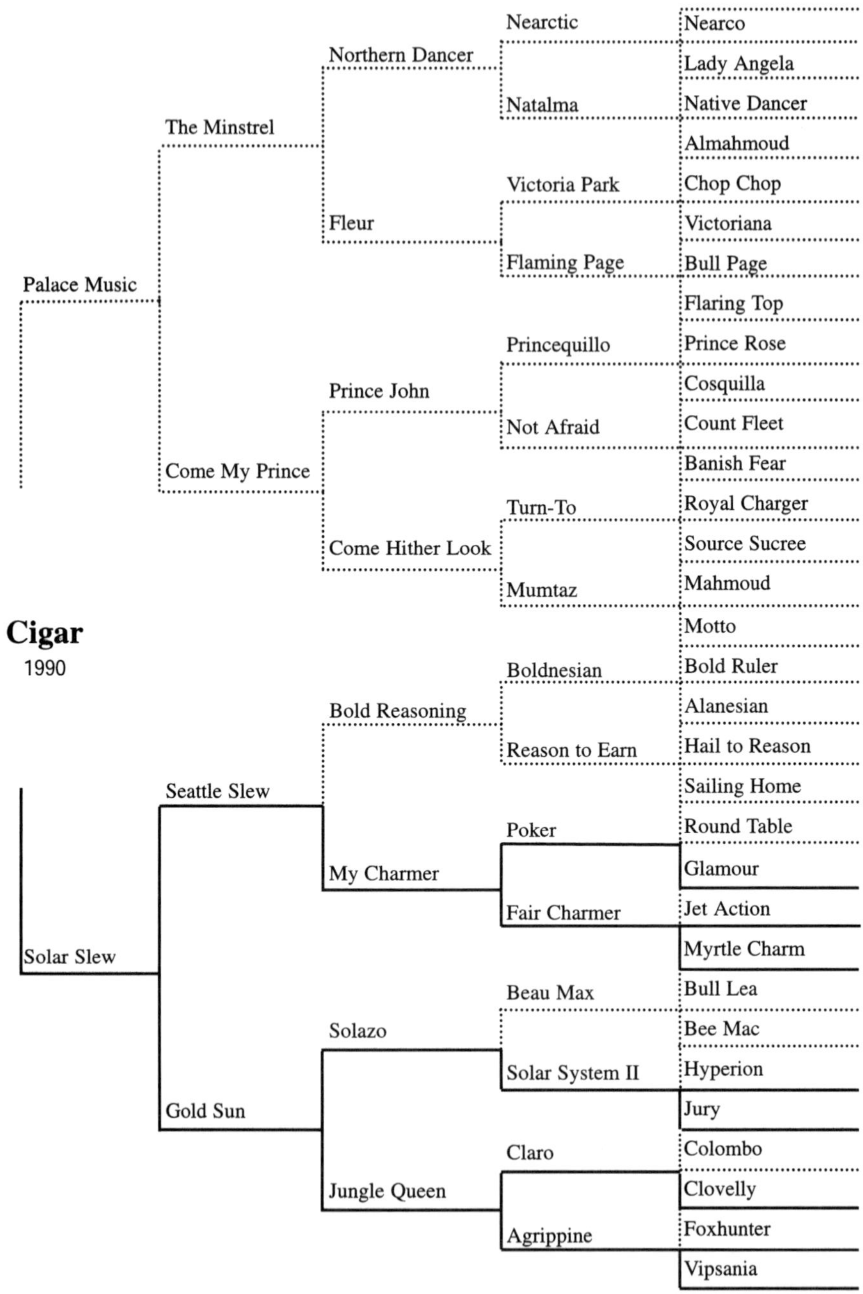
Cigar
1990
Palace Music
The Minstrel
Northern Dancer
Nearctic
Nearco
Lady Angela
Natalma
Native Dancer
Almahmoud
Fleur
Victoria Park
Chop Chop
Victoriana
Flaming Page
Bull Page
Flaring Top
Come My Prince
Prince John
Princequillo
Prince Rose
Cosquilla
Not Afraid
Count Fleet
Banish Fear
Come Hither Look
Turn-To
Royal Charger
Source Sucree
Mumtaz
Mahmoud
Motto
Solar Slew
Seattle Slew
Bold Reasoning
Boldnesian
Bold Ruler
Alanesian
Reason to Earn
Hail to Reason
Sailing Home
My Charmer
Poker
Round Table
Glamour
Fair Charmer
Jet Action
Myrtle Charm
Gold Sun
Solazo
Beau Max
Bull Lea
Bee Mac
Solar System II
Hyperion
Jury
Jungle Queen
Claro
Colombo
Clovelly
Agrippine
Foxhunter
Vipsania

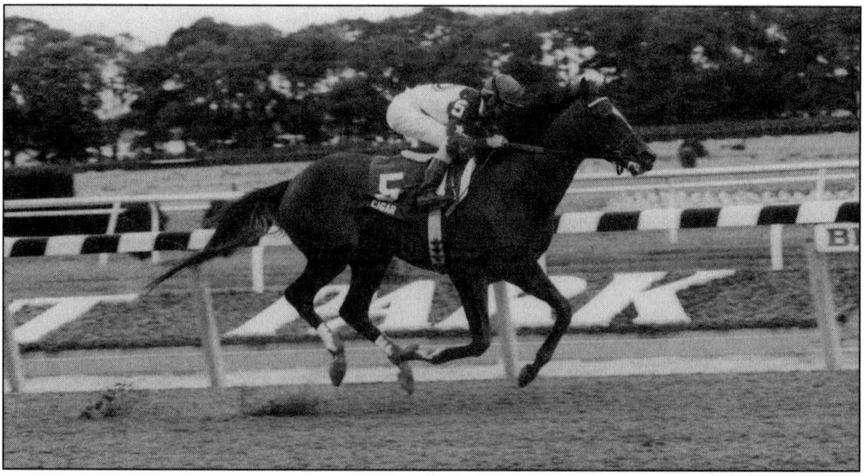

Photo courtesy of Patricia McQueen

Champion racehorse Cigar is an example of a great horse coming from the daughter of a broodmare sire. He carries War Admiral's great heart through his dam Solar Slew and broodmare sire Seattle Slew.

stakes winners. Then they become known as "broodmare sires." Such is the case of Alysheba, a champion racehorse who won the Kentucky Derby and the Breeders' Cup Classic and earned nearly $7 million. He was deemed a failure at stud because he didn't produce sons that could accomplish what he did on the track. Now his daughters, which got his large War Admiral heart, are producing stakes winners.

Occasionally a great horse gets lucky at stud and gets a mare with a heart as large or larger than his. Then the resulting son has the chance of performing as well as his sire. Such was the case for Man 'o War and his son War Admiral, one of the most successful proponents of the large heart in today's pedigrees. War Admiral's dam Brushup was by Sweep, who had a larger heart than Man 'o War. The resulting son went on to win the Triple Crown and to sire daughters that passed on his great heart. That super heart went to such notable champions and sires as Triple Crown winners Affirmed and Seattle Slew, champion Silver Charm, the brilliantly fast champion Dr. Fager, as well as Horse of the Year Buckpasser, Irish champions El Gran Senor and Woodman, champion Real Quiet, Private Account and Fappiano, to name a few.

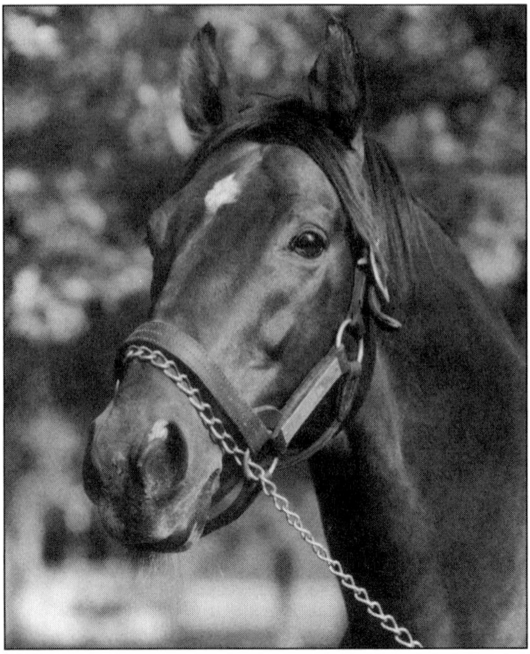

Alysheba is an example of a broodmare sire. Instead of his sons carrying on his accomplishments on the track, it was Alysheba's daughters who gained recognition for producing stakes winners.

Photo courtesy of ***Patricia McQueen***

Those same sires have passed on War Admiral's heart to their daughters, which have performed admirably on the track and have gone on to produce many stakes winners themselves. Through his daughter Solar Slew, Seattle Slew gave War Admiral's great heart to champion Cigar, who tied the record of another great-hearted champion, Citation, when he won 16 races in a row.

While having a large heart in a racehorse is not a guarantee of a winner, it is approximately 25 percent of what makes a champion. In a game where odds count, it behooves the breeder or owner to be sure there is a racing engine that can "go the distance" in his Derby prospect.

Alysheba

1984

Alydar	Raise A Native	Native Dancer	Polynesian	Unbreakable
				Black Polly
			Geisha	Discovery
				Miyako
		Raise You	Case Ace	Teddy
				Sweetheart
			Lady Glory	American Flag
				Beloved
	Sweet Tooth	On-And-On	Nasrullah	Nearco
				Mumtaz Begum
			Two Lea	Bull Lea
				Two Bob
		Plum Cake	Ponder	Pensive
				Miss Rushin
			Real Delight	Bull Lea
				Blue Delight
Bel Sheba	Lt. Stevens	Nantallah	Nasrullah	Nearco
				Mumtaz Begum
			Shimmer	Flares
				Broad Ripple
		Rough Shod II	Gold Bridge	Golden Boss
				Flying Diadem
			Dalmary	Blandford
				Simon's Shoes
	Belthazar	War Admiral	Man 'o War	Fair Play
				Mahubah
			Brushup	Sweep
				Annette K.
		Blinking Owl	Pharamond II	Phalaris
				Selene
			Baba Kenny	Black Servant
				Betty Beall

Weekend Surprise
1980

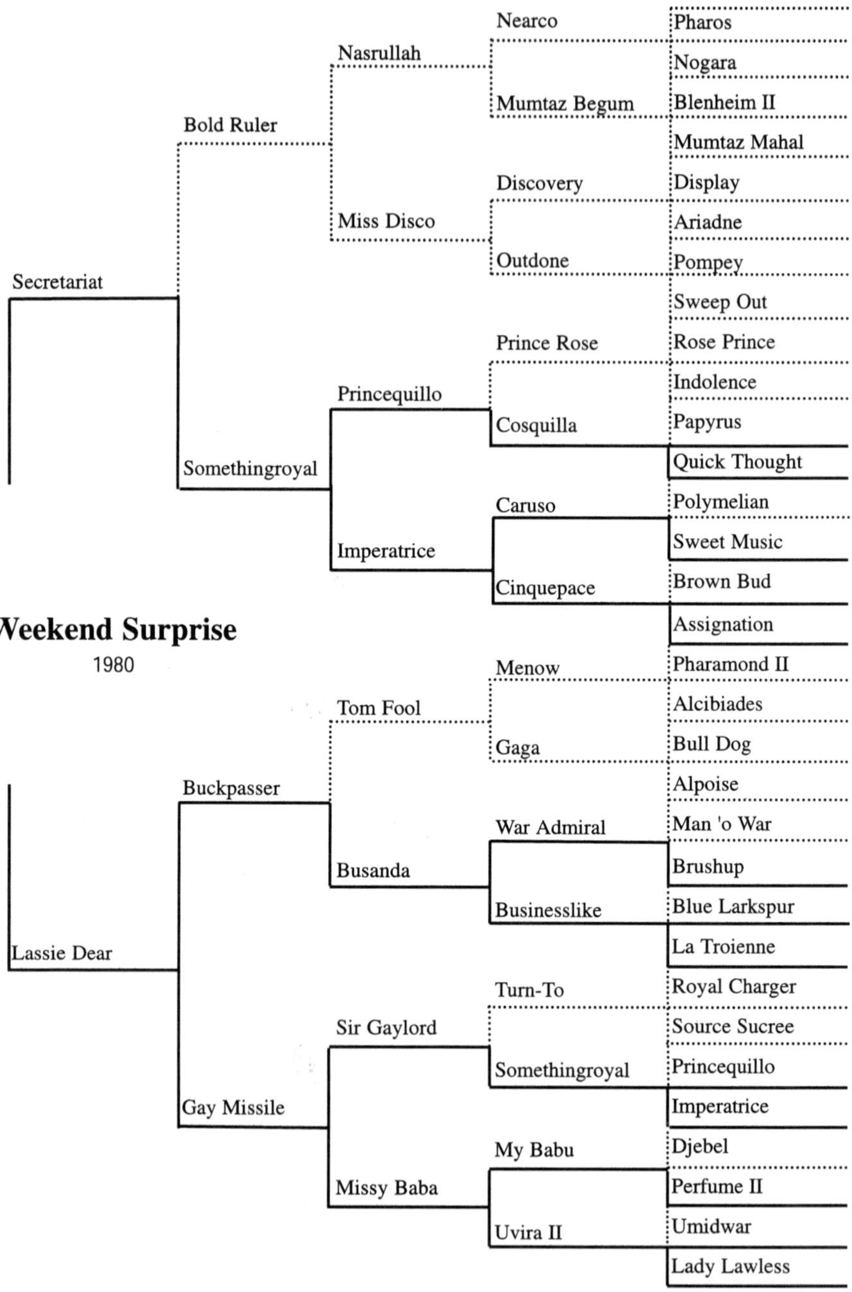

Chapter 7

Double-Copy and Single-Copy Mares

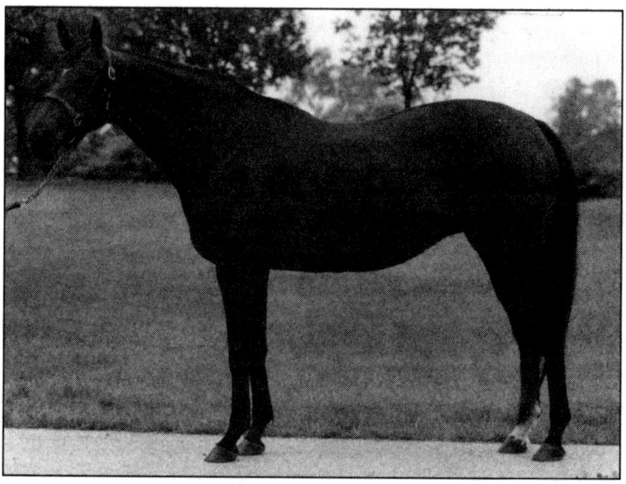

Photo courtesy of Photos by Z

Weekend Surprise (Secretariat x Lassie Dear)

An example of a double-copy mare is the great Thoroughbred broodmare Weekend Surprise, who died after foaling her final daughter in the spring of 2001. A daughter of Secretariat, she was out of a double-copy dam.

Weekend Surprise is among a handful of genetic marvels in the history of Thoroughbred breeding. She had the same Princequillo heart on both of her X chromosomes, one from her sire Secretariat and the other from Sir Gaylord, his half-brother. She was found to have a heart score of 137, which is the score found on the Sir Gaylord heartline. She carried Secretariat's great heart as a recessive. Because she had Princequillo on both Xs, her sons always got the Princequillo X.

Among the horses produced by Weekend Surprise are Horse of the Year A.P. Indy and millionaire Summer Squall. Both sires now are producing outstanding daughters, and when mated with large-hearted mares are producing outstanding sons.

Weekend Surprise's dam Lassie Dear, also a double copy, was by Buckpasser out of Gay Missile by Sir Gaylord. Like her daughter, she produced all winners and she gave the Sir Gaylord X to her daughter. The Sir Gaylord X carries a heart score of 137-140 and has been found repeatedly in horses carrying him on their X line, such as the sire Shelter Half, who is out of a daughter of Sir Gaylord. It was also found by Dr. Fregin in 1974 when he measured fillies and colts at Penny Chenery's The Meadow in Doswell, Virginia. It was discovered in a daughter and a grandson and has been found in measurements we have done in the past six years. It has been amazingly consistent.

The heart scores done at The Meadow in 1974 were only recently discovered by Chenery while going through old files. Among the gems in the measurements was a daughter of Buckpasser, Hatton's Rose, who as a long yearling already had a heart score of 133 which would easily develop into the typical Buckpasser heart score of 147-150. Also among the horses measured that day was the sire First Landing, who had a heart score of 136.

A famous single-copy mare who expressed the large heart but carried the small heart of her sire on her other X chromosome is Kentucky Derby winner Winning Colors. She was measured and found to have the large heart coming from her maternal granddam Miss Carmie, who carried one of the four largest heart lines from the famous broodmare sire Blue Larkspur.

There always will be single-copy mares that expressed the large heart of their sire but carried a small heart from their dam. These mares can perform brilliantly on the track then disappoint in the breeding shed when they are either bred to normal-hearted sires or send the small heart to their sons and daughters.

Winning Colors' sire, Caro, was found at autopsy to have a small- to normal-sized heart. Breeding Winning Colors to a sire with a normal heart size would increase the possibility of her producing a foal with a small to normal heart.

Pocahontas is the most famous example of a broodmare that traced back to the same source of the large heart on both of her X chromosomes. She carried Eclipse's heart from his daughter Everlasting, both through her sire Glencoe and through her tail-female line. It was through the half-sisters Fractious and Fraxinella that she went to that tight gene pool. It is the reason for her being the most important source of Eclipse's heart in the Thoroughbred breed.

Ironically, another great broodmare, La Troienne, found her way to Everlasting on both of her Xs without the benefit of Pocahontas, although she had numerous links to Pocahontas on her bottom side. But the interesting inbreeding in her pedigree was her X line to Sterling, who is found on both the X lines of her sire Teddy and her dam. In La Troienne's pedigree most roads led to Eclipse, some through Pocahontas and two directly to Everlasting through Sterling (found both on the top and bottom of her pedigree).

Foaled in 1868, Sterling was out of a mare named Whisper (1857) who was by Flatcatcher, who had a fascinating tail-female line. Flatcatcher's dam Decoy (1830) was out of Finesse (1815), who was out of Violante by John Bull, whose dam Xantippe was by Eclipse. Violante was out of a daughter of Highflyer simply known as Highflyer mare, that was out of Everlasting by Eclipse.

Whisper's bottom side is very interesting as well. Her dam was Silence, foaled in 1848 by Melbourne. Melbourne is out of a daughter of Cervantes, who is out of Evelina by Highflyer. The Cervantes daughter is out of a Golumpus mare out of a Pavnator mare out of a St. George mare. St. George is out of a daughter of Eclipse.

It doesn't stop there. Silence's dam has an interesting tail-female line as well. Her dam Secret was foaled in 1841. Secret's fourth dam is Cobbea by Skyscraper, who is by Highflyer and out of Everlasting by Eclipse. There is definitely a pattern here and Eclipse is the key.

Pocahontas

1837

Glencoe	Sultan	Selim	Buzzard	Woodpecker
				Misfortune
			Alexander Mare	Alexander
				Highflyer Mare
		Bacchante	Williamson's Ditto	Sir Peter
				Arethusa
			Mercury Mare	Mercury
				Herod Mare
	Trampoline	Tramp	Dick Andrews	Joe Andrews
				Highflyer Mare
			Gohanna Mare	Gohanna
				Fraxinella
		Web	Waxy	Pot-8-O's
				Maria
			Penelope	Trumpator
				Prunella
Marpessa	Muley	Orville	Beningbrough	King Fergus
				Herod B. Mare
			Evelina	Highflyer
				Termagant
		Eleanor	Whiskey	Saltram
				Calash
			Young Giantess	Diomed
				Giantess
	Clare	Marmion	Whiskey	Saltram
				Calash
			Y. Giantess	Diomed
				Giantess
		Hapalice	Gohanna	Mercury
				Dr. Of Herod
			Amazon	Driver
				Fractious

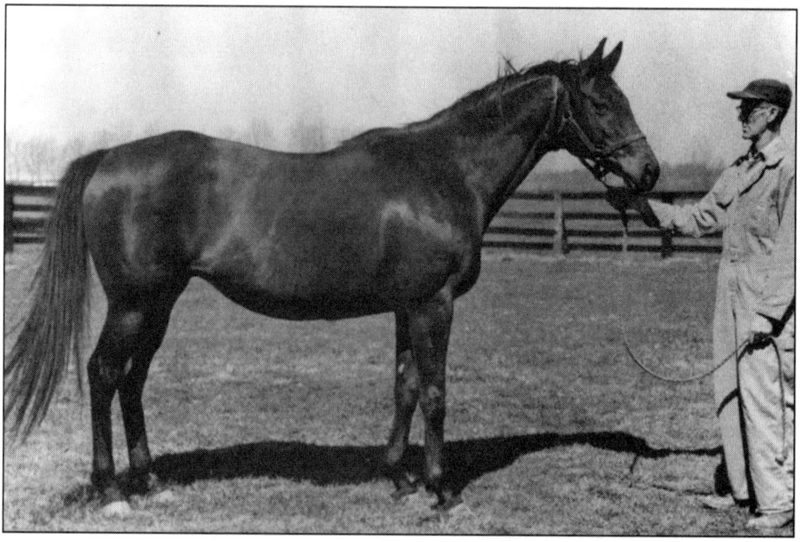

Photo courtesy of Keeneland Library/J.C. Skeets Meadors

Striking, a daughter of War Admiral

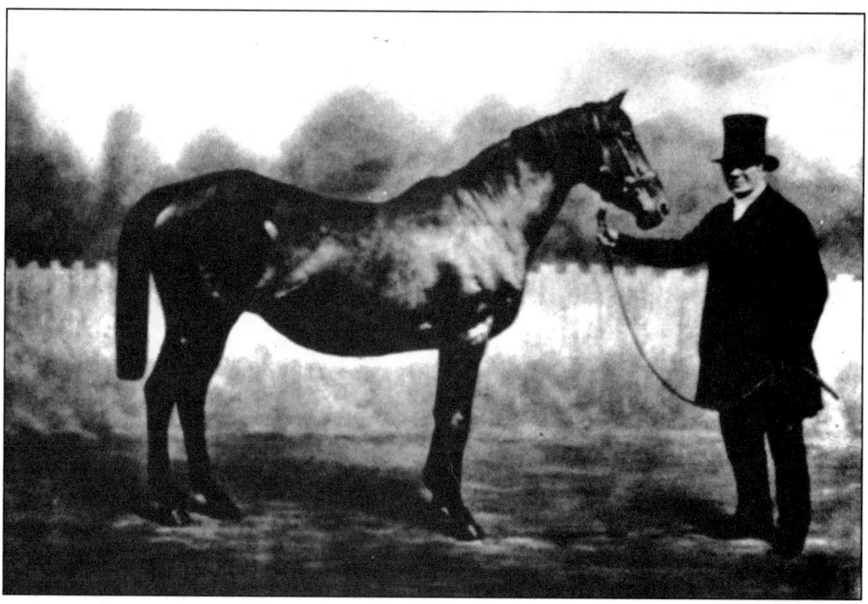

Photo courtesy of Grayson/Sutcliffe Collection

Pocahontas (Glencoe x Marpessa), who carries Eclipse's heart

La Troienne
1926

Teddy	Ajax	Flying Fox	Orne	Ormonde
				Angelica
			Vampire	Galopin
				Irony
		Amie	Clamart	Saumur
				Princess Catherine
			Alice	Wellingtonia
				Asta
	Rondeau	Bay Ronald	Hampton	Lord Clifden
				Lady Langden
			Black Duchess	Galliard
				Black Corrie
		Doremi	Bend Or	Doncaster
				Rouge Rose
			Lady Emily	Macaroni
				May Queen
Helene De Troie	Helicon	Cyllene	Bona Vista	Bend Or
				Vista
			Arcadia	Isonomy
				Distant Shore
		Vain Duchess	Isinglass	Isonomy
				Deadlock
			Sweet Duchess	Hagioscope
				Grand Duchess
	Lady of Pedigree	St. Denis	St. Simon	Galopin
				St. Angela
			Brooch	Blue-Green
				Ornament
		Doxa	Melton	Master Kildare
				Violet Melrose
			Paradoxical	Timothy
				Inchbonny

Another outstanding double-copy mare in the mold of Pocahontas, Weekend Surprise and La Troienne is My Charmer, dam of Seattle Slew. My Charmer traces to two full sisters on her X lines. Both are daughters of War Admiral out of daughters of Bubbling Over, who passes the Sweep heart, the source of War

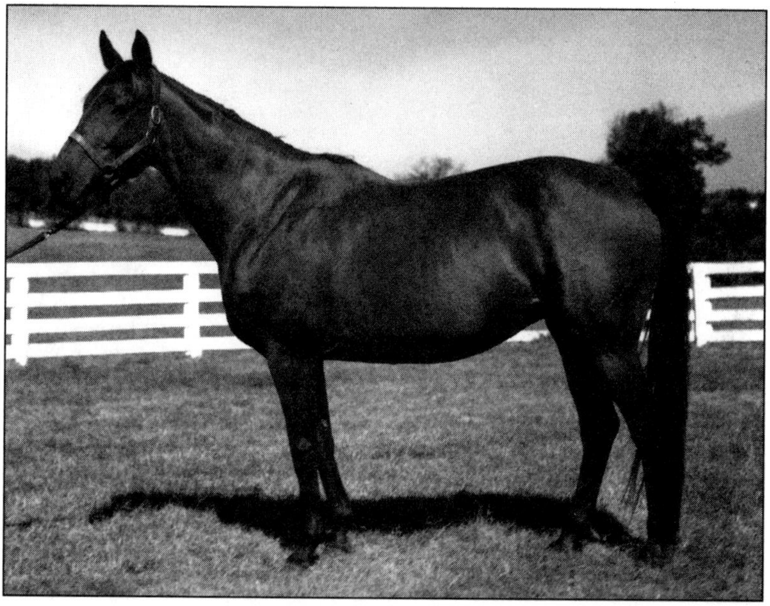

Photo courtesy of the Grayson/Sutcliffe Collection

La Troienne (Teddy x Helene De Troie)

Admiral's heart. This is the same tight gene pool found in the other mares that increases their odds of passing the same heart to all offspring. All of My Charmer's sons have produced great daughters. My Charmer gave Poker's heart to Seattle Slew, which comes from War Admiral's daughter Striking, who turned out to be a better producer than her sister Busher. There is a strong resemblance in the daughters of Seattle Slew who express his X. This same resemblance is seen in Desert Secret's daughters like Tale of Two Hearts, who received the My Charmer X from Desert Secret. Horses expressing this X seem to have a similar body type, large feet and reactive personalities.

My Charmer

1969

- Poker
  - Round Table
    - Princequillo
      - Prince Rose
        - Rose Prince
        - Indolence
      - Cosquilla
        - Papyrus
        - Quick Thought
    - Knight's Daughter
      - Sir Cosmo
        - The Boss
        - Ayn Hali
      - Feola
        - Friar Marcus
        - Aloe
  - Glamour
    - Nasrullah
      - Nearco
        - Pharos
        - Nogara
      - Mumtaz Begum
        - Blenheim
        - Mumtaz Mahal
    - Striking
      - War Admiral
        - Man 'o War
        - Brushup
      - Baby League
        - Bubbling Over
        - La Troienne
- Fair Charmer
  - Jet Action
    - Jet Pilot
      - Blenheim II
        - Blandford
        - Malva
      - Black Wave
        - Sir Gallahad
        - Black Curl
    - Busher
      - War Admiral
        - Man 'o War
        - Brushup
      - Baby League
        - Bubbling Over
        - La Troienne
  - Myrtle Charm
    - Alsab
      - Good Goods
        - Neddie
        - Brocatelle
      - Winds Chant
        - Wildair
        - Eulogy
    - Crepe Myrtle
      - Equipoise
        - Pennant
        - Swinging
      - Myrtlewood
        - Blue Larkspur
        - Frizeur

When it comes to identifying double-copy mares, it is important to look at the pattern of performance in their produce. As stated earlier, an excellent guide is to look at the male offspring of mares. When considering younger mares that have no offspring, then the pedigree, conformation and performance record must be your guide.

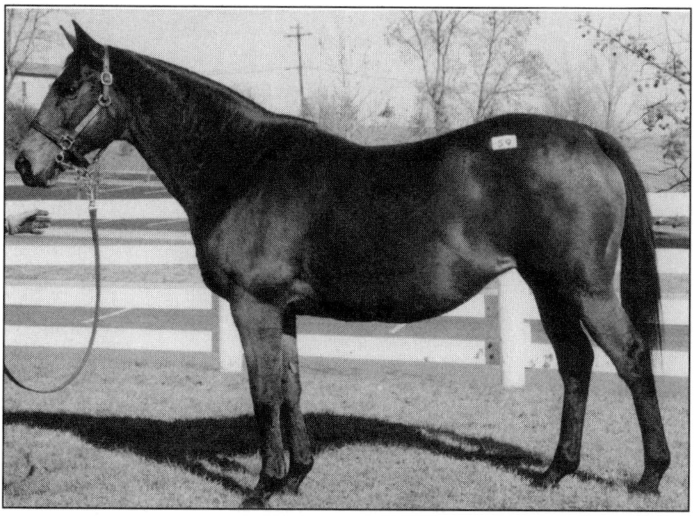

Photo courtesy of The Thoroughbred Times

My Charmer, dam of Seattle Slew, is another example of a successful double-copy mare.

It is important to measure your broodmare so you know for sure what kind of heart she is carrying and capable of passing on to half of her offspring. It is hard to identify double-copy mares without years of measuring offspring unless they are by a sire whose heart score you already know and they express the bottom side of their pedigree. This is always seen as a gift. It is that recessive or hidden X that is so hard to identify.

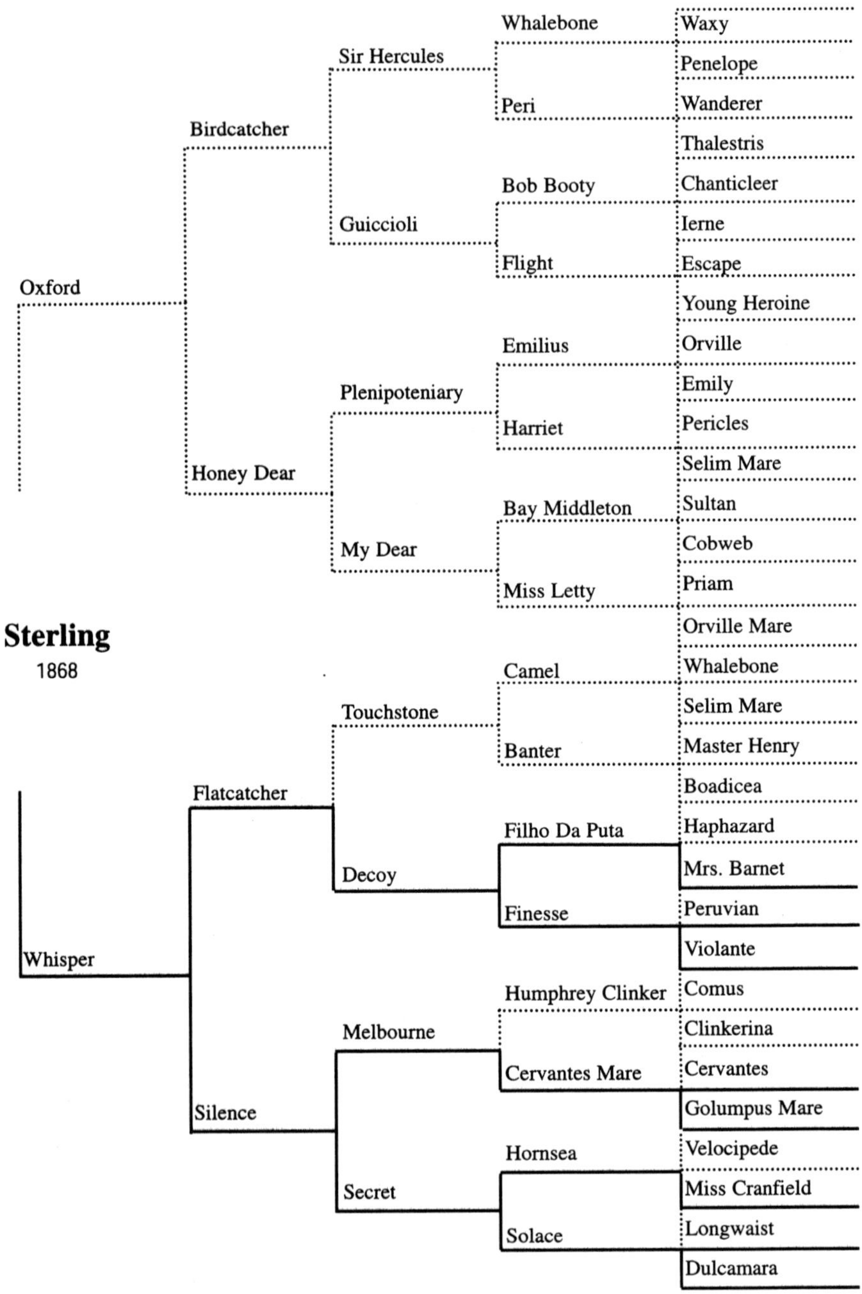
Sterling
1868
Oxford
Birdcatcher
Sir Hercules
Whalebone
Waxy
Penelope
Peri
Wanderer
Thalestris
Guiccioli
Bob Booty
Chanticleer
Ierne
Flight
Escape
Young Heroine
Honey Dear
Plenipoteniary
Emilius
Orville
Emily
Harriet
Pericles
Selim Mare
My Dear
Bay Middleton
Sultan
Cobweb
Miss Letty
Priam
Orville Mare
Whisper
Flatcatcher
Touchstone
Camel
Whalebone
Selim Mare
Banter
Master Henry
Boadicea
Decoy
Filho Da Puta
Haphazard
Mrs. Barnet
Finesse
Peruvian
Violante
Silence
Melbourne
Humphrey Clinker
Comus
Clinkerina
Cervantes Mare
Cervantes
Golumpus Mare
Secret
Hornsea
Velocipede
Miss Cranfield
Solace
Longwaist
Dulcamara

Double-Copy Thoroughbred Mares*

Adoryphar
Alcibiades
Alluvial
Almahmoud
Althea
Araucaria
Aspidistra
Aura of Glory
Baby League
Bathing Girl
Bee Mac
Be Faithful
Bel Sheba
Belthazar
Betty's Secret
Bird Flower
Black Helen
Bloodroot
Blue Banner
Blue Denim
Boat
Bonnie's Poker
Boudoir II
Bramalea
Bright Candles
Broadway
Broadway Boogie
Brushup
Busanda
Busher
Businesslike
C'est Moi Cheri
Cadillacing
Cap and Bells
Carriette
Chalk Box
Chapel of Dreams
Charette
Charming Lassie
Cheerily
Christmas Bonus
Con Game
Cosmah
Cosquilla
Count the Votes
Courtly Dee
Crimson Saint
Cue
Dry North
Duty Dance
East of the Moon
Emerald Reef
Escena
Eternally
Fairy Garden
Falconese
Fall Aspen
Flaming Page
Flanders
Flitabout
Flower Bowl
Fly North
Forever After
Gaga
Gana Facil
Gay Missle
Gertruc Mc
Glorious Song
Golden Ballet
Happy Holme
Heaven Knows Why
Hopespringseternal
Image of Glory
Imperatrice
In Prime Time
Inside Information
In the Curl
Jancy
K D Princess
Katambra
Kerala
Key Bridge
Key Witness
Killaloe
Lady Angela
Lady Josephine
Lady's Secret
Lady Windborne
Lassie Dear
La Troienne
Lovage
Mah Mahal
Maplejinsky
Miesque
Milan Mill
Millicent
Minnette
Miss Carmie
Miss Zigby
Misty Morn
Mocassin
Moscow Tap
Moscow TV
Mumtaz Begum
Mumtaz Mahal

My Charmer
My Dear Girl
My Flag
Myrtlewood
Natalma
Naval Orange
Never Hula
Never Knock
Noble Lassie
Northern Sunset
Numbered Account
Passing Mood
Personal Ensign
Planting Time
Plucky Liege
Political Favor
Prayer Bell
Pure Profit
Quickly
Raise an Heiress
Rare Mint
Relaxing
River Fairy
Romanella
Rough Shod II
Saintly Manner
Secrettame
Selene
Sequence
Sewing Lady
Sharon Brown
Shayne McQuire
Shenanigans
Shy Dawn
Sissy's Time
Six Crowns
Soaring Softly
Solar Slew
Somethingroyal
South Ocean
Soviet Problem
Special
St. Adele
St. Diva
Strawberry Reason
Strike a Balance
Striking
Sun Colony
Sun Princessa
Sunline
Sunset Wells
Sweet Tooth
Surfside
Talamanca
Tale of Two Hearts
Teleran
Tamerett
Teresa Mc
Terlingua
The Last Red
Time to Plant
Toll Booth
Torelia
Trifecta Box
Wac
Wavy Navy
Wayage
Weekend in Seattle
Weekend Surprise
Welcome Surprise
Won't Tell You
Work the Crowd

** This list is not complete but serves as a guide to mares of the past and present that are found in pedigrees that have passed the tests of time or measurement and are considered to be double-copy mares.*

Chapter 8

Physical Clues to Genetic Traits

In the past six years of research on the X Factor by myself and Dr. Fregin, it is hard not to notice family line characteristics that seem to follow the X line. The most notable of these, which was first noticed by Secretariat's breeder Penny Chenery, is that small ears seem to follow the big heart.

Chenery first noticed a resemblance between Secretariat's small curly ears and those of The Last Red, the twin used in the breeding research. Both horses express the Princequillo X chromosome, Secretariat from his dam Somethingroyal, a daughter of Princequillo, and The Last Red from her sire Moscow Ballet, who gets it from his second dam Milan Mill, another daughter of Princequillo.

In doing photo comparisons with the two horses, one can see that they do have the small curly ears associated with Princequillo. In addition, they have a similar hip, eye and nostrils.

Chenery made this observation while being interviewed for the first X Factor book. Subsequently, we have started following the ears of different lines and have found this method to be amazingly accurate. If a horse inherits a specific ear, he gets the same heart score. Geneticist Dr. Gus Cothran of the University of Kentucky believes that the ears are a physical marker for a genetic trait on the X chromosome inherited by the horse.

While discerning the differences in ears would take an artist's eye in most cases, there is a specific ear on one of the four great heartlines that is easy to spot - the small rounded ear of Mahmoud. When viewed from the front, the ear has a leaf-like quality which is unmistakable. Northern Dancer and Halo had this ear. Spectacular Bid also has this round ear as does Machiavellian, who stands in England.

Fusiachi Pegasus inherited these small round ears, courtesy of Halo, the sire of his maternal granddam Rowdy Angel, along with Mahmoud's great heart and it helped enable him to win the Kentucky Derby in 2000. He was a record yearling, bringing $4 million at Keeneland. But he ended up a Derby winner with earnings of more than $1.9 million and was sold for stud for a reported whopping figure between $60 million and $70 million.

With Approval, whose dam Passing Mood was by Buckpasser out of Cool Mood by Northern Dancer out of Happy Mood by Mahmoud, has the small round ears and a body that looks very much like Mahmoud's. Passing Mood obviously gave him the Mahmoud X.

Interestingly enough, she had another famous son, Touch Gold, to whom she gave the Buckpasser X. He looked nothing like With Approval but very much like the Buckpasser-line stallions. His ears are the medium sculptured ears of the War Admiral line, and his body type is also of that line.

Those funny ears can come up the female line from a long way off. In the case of Silver Deputy, who also has the small round ears, they came up his tail-female line from a daughter of Gallant Man, who carried the Mahmoud X. Silver Deputy has been successful in passing that large Mahmoud heart on to his daughters.

It has become a shortcut — and an amazingly accurate one — for us in measuring horses to check the ears and compare the heart score after the horse has been measured. Just as humans look for family resemblances in their offspring, seeking physical similarities in foals is a clue to which X has been expressed.

There are always choices. In the case of a filly that inherits two X chromosomes, she can be influenced by either her sire or her dam. It is a matter of which X is dominant and which is expressed. She will carry the other X as a recessive and be able to pass it off to 50 percent of her offspring.

With a colt, it is a matter of determining which of his dam's two Xs he inherited. Whichever X, that will be his expressed heart and the X he will give to all of his daughters.

With the Alysheba colt out of The Last Red, he has Man 'o War's ears with a distinctive notch on them and his front end with its distinctive withers. In looking at conformation shots of Man 'o War and his descendants that express his X chromosome, there is a striking resemblance in the front end and withers of these horses. Man 'o War had high, pronounced withers with a rounded appearance that reminds me of a "dowager's hump." His front end had an upright appearance, although he was by no means straight-shouldered. It was a powerful shoulder and very distinctive. When comparing conformation photographs of Man 'o War, his dam Mahubah, her sire Rock Sand and Man 'o War's daughters, as well as other descendants such as Spotted Bull, Hempen, Spy Song and Coup de Cas, there is a very strong family resemblance. The Man 'o War front end and rounded withers are easy to spot and obviously follow the X chromosome trail.

Mahmoud

1933

- Blenheim II
  - Blandford
    - Swynford
      - John O'Gaunt
        - Isinglass
        - La Fleche
      - Canterbury Pilgrim
        - Tristan
        - Pilgrimage
    - Blanche
      - White Eagle
        - Gallinule
        - Merry Gal
      - Black Cherry
        - Bendigo
        - Black Duchess
  - Malva
    - Charles O'Malley
      - Desmond
        - St. Simon
        - L'abese De Jouarre
      - Goody Two Shoes
        - Isinglass
        - Sandal II
    - Wild Arum
      - Robert Le Diable
        - Ayrshire
        - Rose Bay
      - Marliacea
        - Martagon
        - Flitters
- Mah Mahal
  - Gainsborough
    - Bayardo
      - Bay Ronald
        - Hampton
        - Black Duchess
      - Galicia
        - Galopin
        - Isoletta
    - Rosedrop
      - St. Frusquin
        - St. Simon
        - Isabel
      - Rosaline
        - Trenton
        - Rosalys
  - Mumtaz Mahal
    - The Tetrarch
      - Roi Herode
        - Le Samaritain
        - Roxelane
      - Vahren
        - Bona Vista
        - Castania
    - Lady Josephine
      - Sundridge
        - Amphion
        - Sierra
      - Americus Girl
        - Americus
        - Palotta

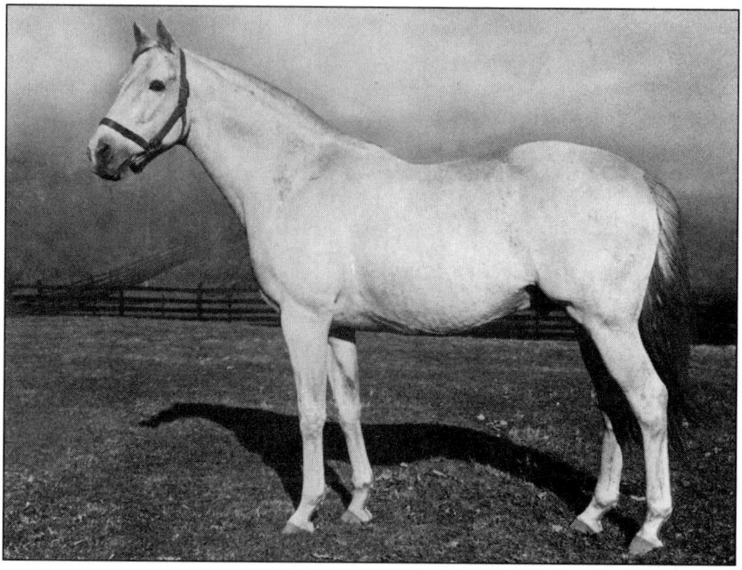

Photo courtesy of the Keeneland Library/J.C. Skeets Meadors

Mahmoud (Blenheim II x Mah Mahal),
whose small rounded ears can be seen in his descendants.

Northern Dancer

1961

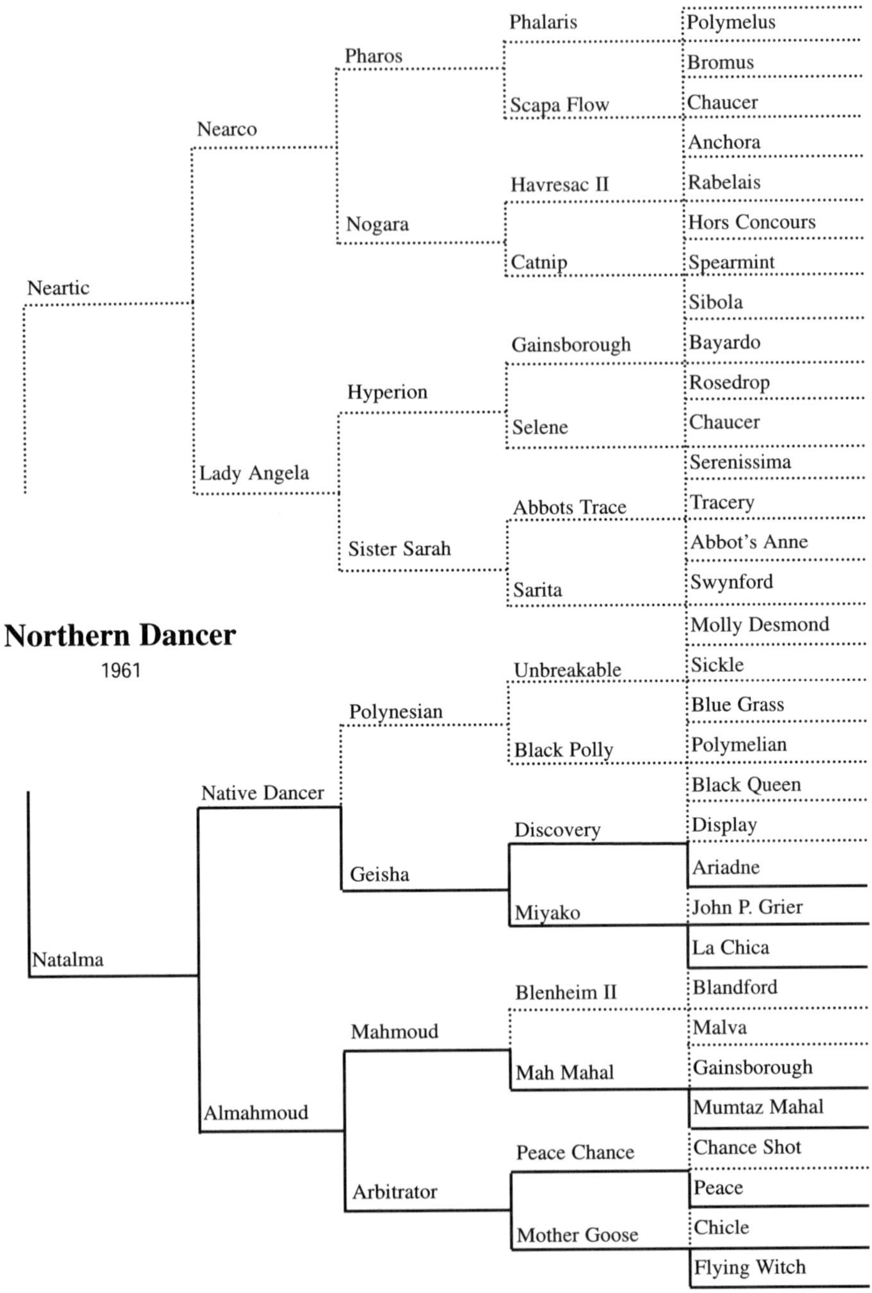

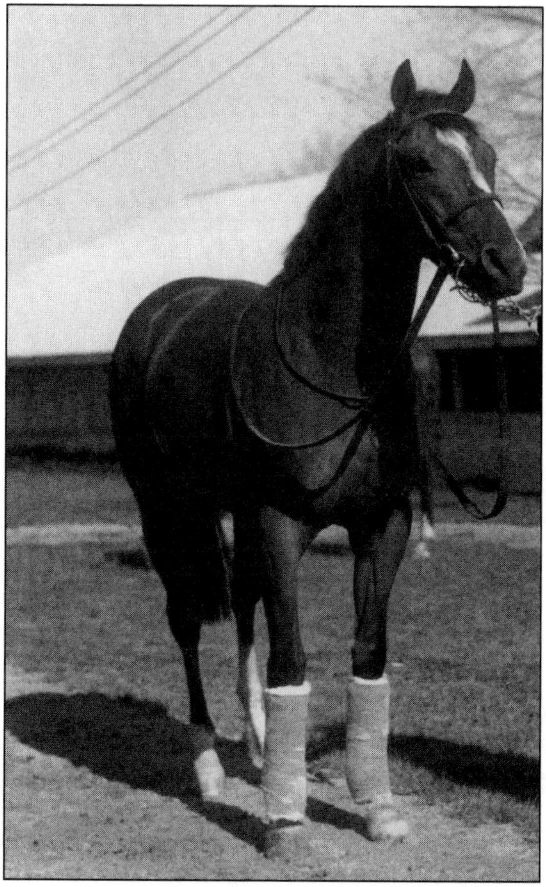

Photo courtesy of the Thoroughbred Times

Northern Dancer (Nearctic x Natalma),
who carries the Mahmoud X.

With Approval

1986

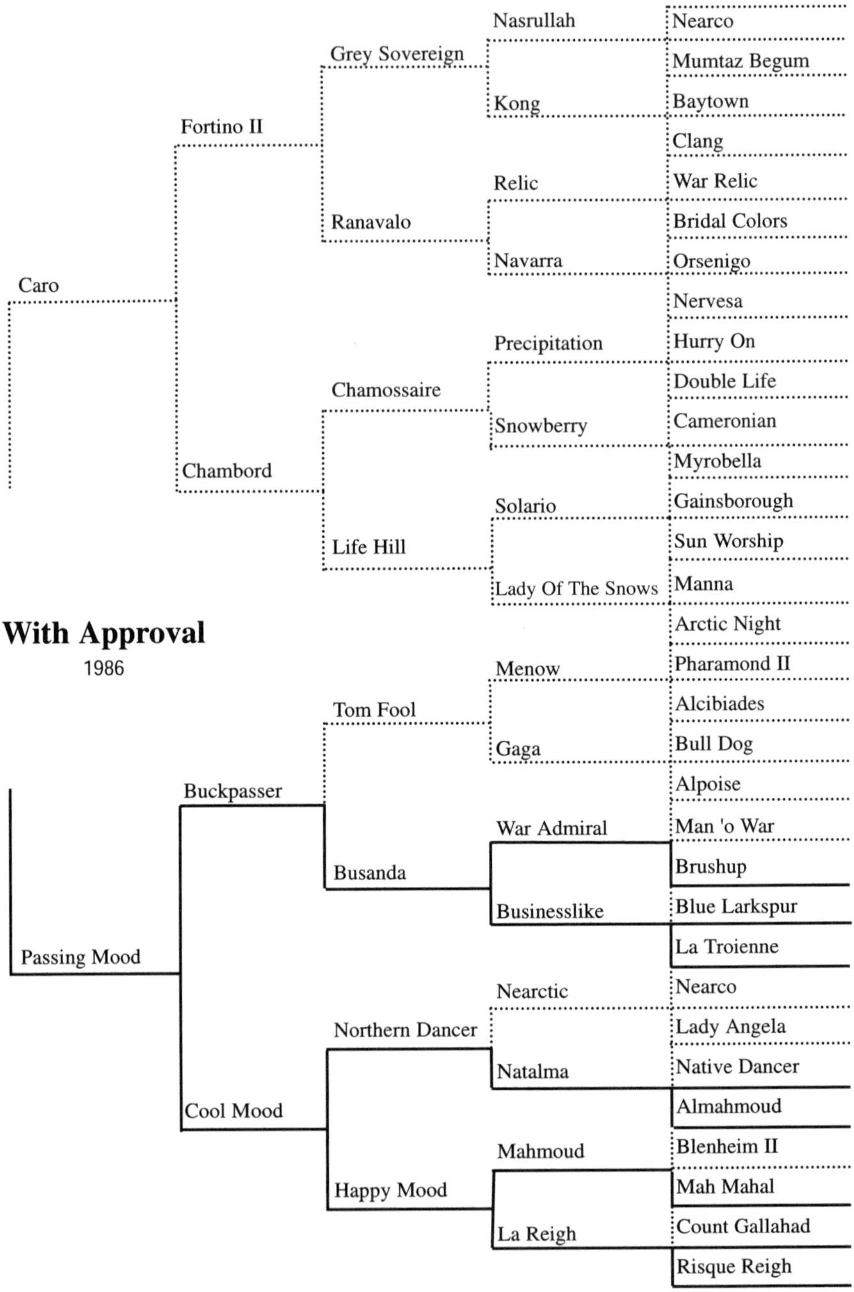

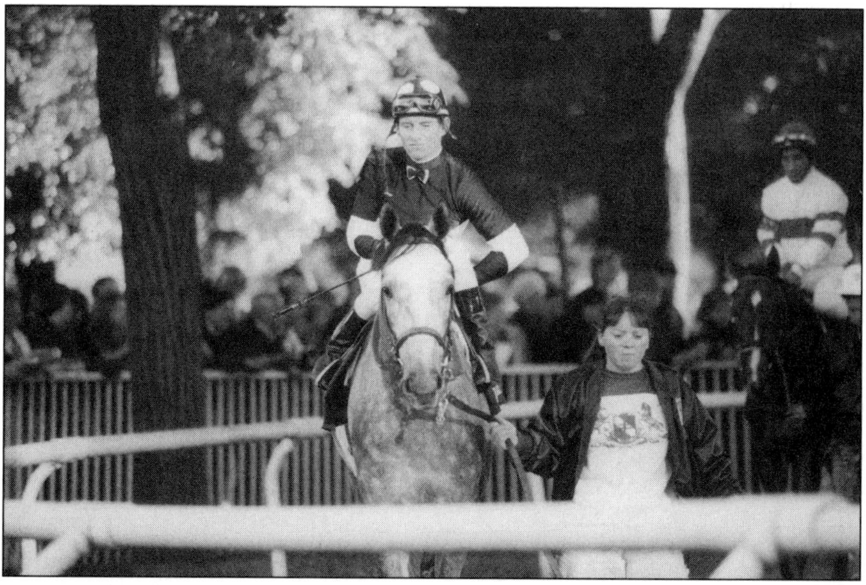

Photo courtesy of the Thoroughbred Times

With Approval

Halo

1969

- Hail to Reason
  - Turn-To
    - Royal Charger
      - Nearco
        - Pharos
        - Nogara
      - Sun Princess
        - Solario
        - Mumtaz Begum
    - Source Sucree
      - Admiral Drake
        - Craig An Eran
        - Plucky Liege
      - Lavendula
        - Pharos
        - Sweet Lavender
  - Nothirdchance
    - Blue Swords
      - Blue Larkspur
        - Black Servant
        - Blossom Time
      - Flaming Swords
        - Man 'o War
        - Exalted
    - Galla Colors
      - Sir Gallahad III
        - Teddy
        - Plucky Liege
      - Rouge et Noir
        - St. Germany
        - Baton Rouge
- Cosmah
  - Cosmic Bomb
    - Pharamond II
      - Phalaris
        - Polymelus
        - Bromus
      - Selene
        - Chaucer
        - Serenissima
    - Banish Fear
      - Blue Larkspur
        - Black Servant
        - Blossom Time
      - Herodiade
        - Over There
        - Herodias
  - Almahmoud
    - Mahmoud
      - Blenheim II
        - Blandford
        - Malva
      - Mah Mahal
        - Gainsborough
        - Mumtaz Mahal
    - Arbitrator
      - Peace Chance
        - Chance Shot
        - Peace
      - Mother Goose
        - Chicle
        - Flying Witch

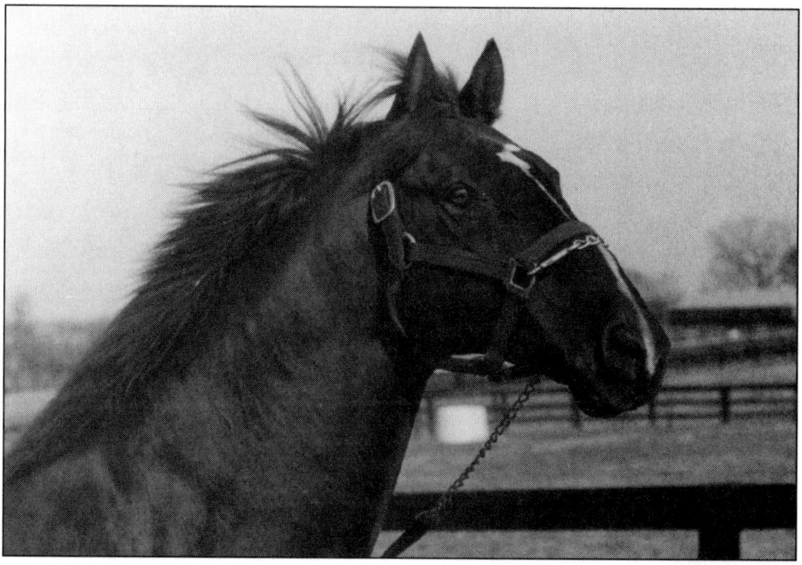

Photo courtesy of Photos by Z

Halo
(Hail To Reason x Cosmah)

Fusaichi Pegasus

1997

Mr. Prospector	Raise A Native	Native Dancer	Polynesian	Unbreakable
				Black Polly
			Geisha	Discovery
				Miyako
		Raise You	Case Ace	Teddy
				Sweetheart
			Lady Glory	American Flag
				Beloved
	Gold Digger	Nashua	Nasrullah	Nearco
				Mumtaz Begum
			Segula	Johnstown
				Sekhmet
		Sequence	Count Fleet	Reigh Count
				Quickly
			Miss Dogwood	Bull Dog
				Myrtlewood
Angel Fever	Danzig	Northern Dancer	Nearctic	Nearco
				Lady Angela
			Natalma	Native Dancer
				Almahmoud
		Pas de Nom	Admiral's Voyage	Crafty Admiral
				Olympia Lou
			Petitioner	Petition
				Steady Aim
	Rowdy Angel	Halo	Hail to Reason	Turn-to
				Nothirdchance
			Cosmah	Cosmic Bomb
				Almahmoud
		Ramhyde	Rambunctious	Rasper II
				Danae II
			Castle Hyde	Tulyar
				Bold Irish

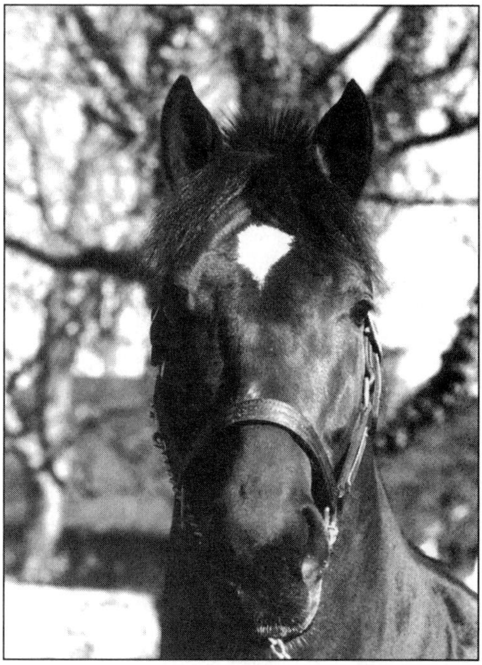

Photo courtesy of Marianna Haun

Fusiachi Pegasus

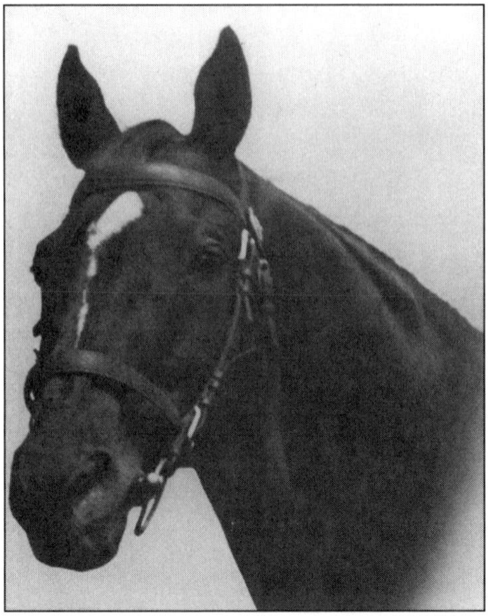

Photo courtesy of the Grayson/Sutcliffe Collection

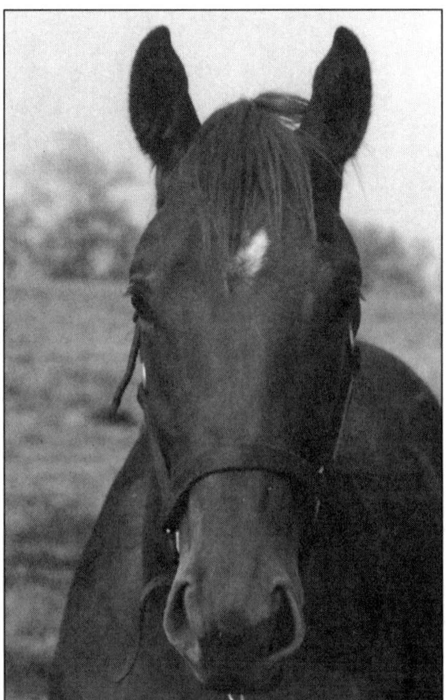

Photo courtesy of Marianna Haun

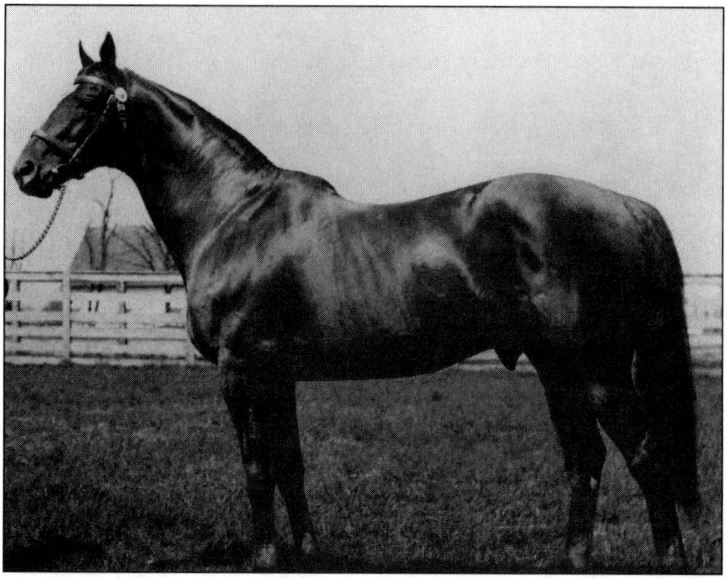

Photo courtesy of the Grayson/Sutcliffe Collection

The photos on these two pages show the physical resemblances among Man 'o War and his descendants. Pictured are Man 'o War (above) and Spotted Bull (below), and Man 'o War (preceding page, top) and Man 'o Sheba. The distinctive Man 'o War ears are visible here, while Spotted Bull also portrays his high, rounded and powerful withers.

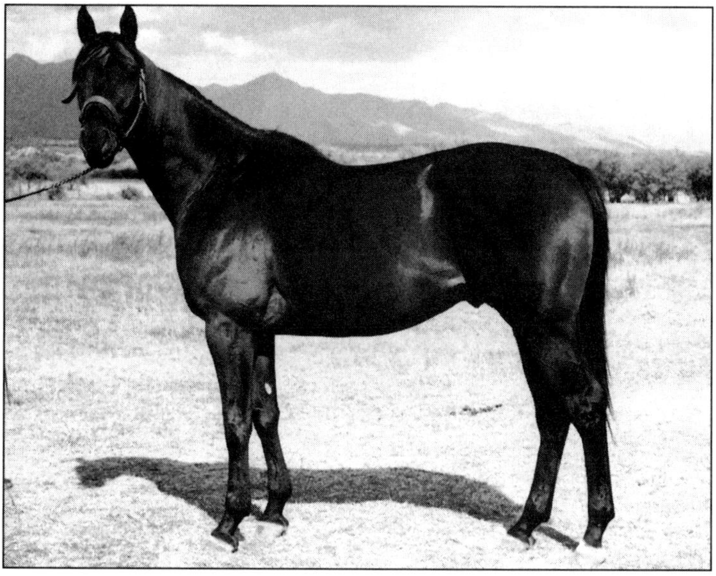

Photo courtesy of the American Quarter Horse Association

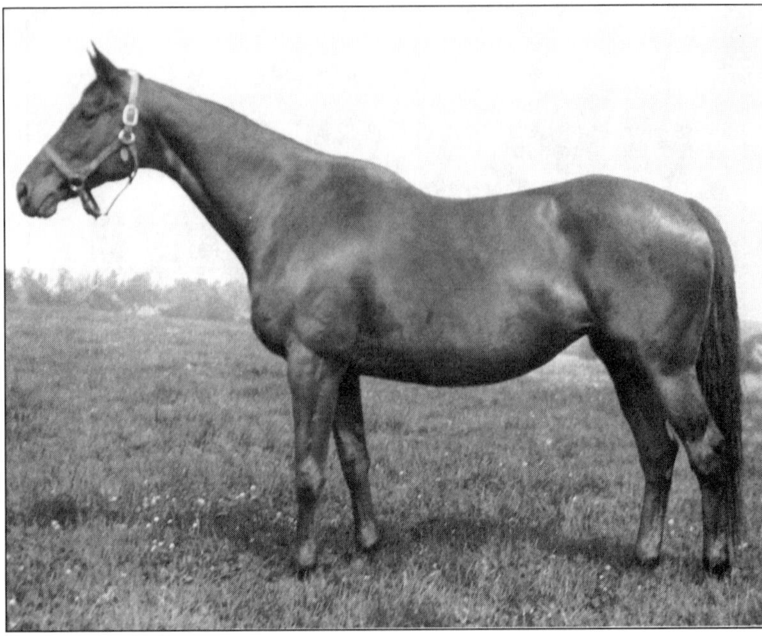

Photos courtesy of the Grayson/Sutcliffe Collection

Mahubah, dam of Man 'o War (top)
and Mata Hari, granddaughter of Man 'o War

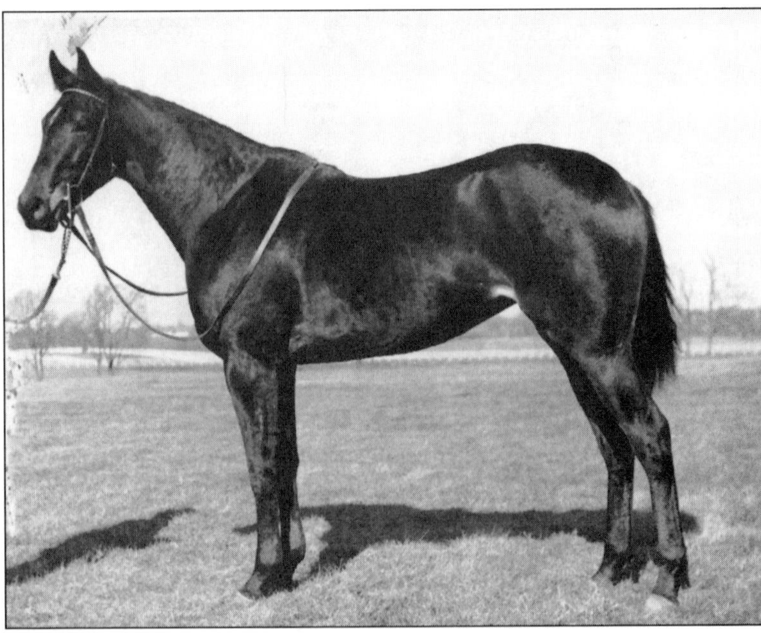

Chapter 9

Looking For the Great Heart

In trying to breed superior individuals, it is important to know what genetic tools you are working with in today's pedigrees. You need to understand which individuals are passing great heart, which are passing brilliant speed and which combine the two elements.

Because most stud farms would object to someone showing up with an ECG machine to test their stallions, it is important to look for clues in the horses' pedigrees and performance on the track. The stud book can be a very useful tool. It can tell you more than most people are aware.

The first thing to look for is a pattern of performance on the X line, particularly where it gives the produce of the dams in the pedigree. If a mare's record shows that she has produced 10 runners and 10 winners, that is a pretty good indication that she is probably a double-copy mare. If it says she has 10 runners and five winners, that is the pattern of a single-copy mare. There are always exceptions where an individual's offspring didn't make it on the track because of injury, finances or poor training. Because these things are out of the mare's control, there will be those double-copy mares that had 10 runners and eight winners. But as a rule of thumb, a good produce record indicates a pretty good X being passed.

When looking at a sire's produce, examine his daughters. They are the only ones his heart can influence. When looking at the females on his bottom side look at their sons, which can only be influenced by them. When you see female family members with outstanding sons, you are on to something.

Check the sire's record on the track. How far did he run? If he was basically a sprinter and had better sons than daughters, then he could be a speed sire. This is useful information. If you breed to a speed sire, you want to make sure that you bring to him a mare that not only has speed but also the heart to give to his offspring so they can go the distance. When you are looking at a sire with plenty of heart that has successfully competed at classic distances, you want to make sure you bring him a mare with speed and heart to maximize your options in the offspring.

Because there is no way of controlling which X comes out of a mating, it is important to cover your bases in terms of the choices. It's like developing your own recipe where you combine particular ingredients in hopes of producing an award-winning entrée. You fold in the heart, but don't forget to add a dash of speed. You consider body types. There is the classic long, elegant type that is associated with distance racing and the shorter-coupled more muscular type that is aligned with sprinters. The ideal should be a combination of the two like Secretariat, who had great length of stride, powerful muscles, amazing speed, and the world's greatest heart.

It isn't easy to find the correct combination because so often they seem to be one or the other — distance or speed. If you take a top stallion with one or the other features, you have to provide a mare that can make up what is missing.

In looking at stallions in the Bluegrass in 2001, I found one that I liked in Victory Speech. He had a pattern of performance, earning more than $1.2 million, including the $500,000 Strub Stakes (G1) at four. He had made 27 starts, demonstrating a soundness frequently missing in many of today's sires. He expressed the Alydar X, giving him the Blue Larkspur heart. His Y line was good with a great speed sire in Deputy Minister, a son of Vice Regent — a line that had worked well with my mare before. He was a beautifully made individual with a lovely head and wonderful shoulder. He was also in keeping with my pocketbook.

Unfortunately for me, I picked a bad year in the Bluegrass and my mare was caught up in the problems associated with the

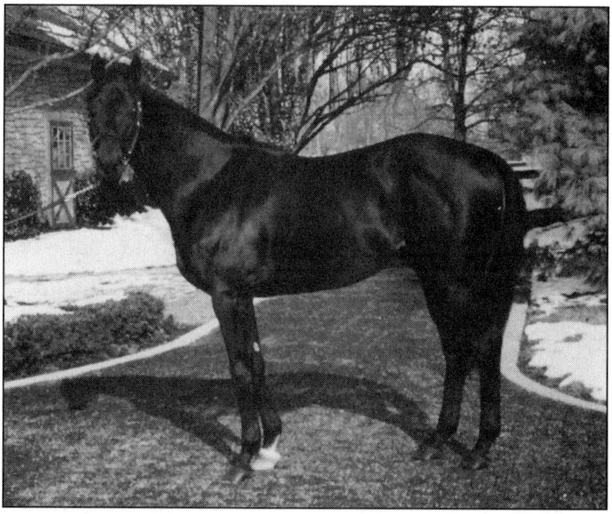

Victory Speech

Photo courtesy of Marianna Haun

foal loss syndrome and refused to develop a breedable follicle. Hopefully, the next year would be better and I could see what this cross might bring. It just goes to show that as Robert Burns said so many years ago, "the best-laid plans of mice and men" can go awry. But when you are trying to breed racehorses in such an expensive business, research is always important and if it doesn't help one year, it can the next.

While the four most successful super-heart lines found in today's pedigrees are Princequillo, War Admiral, Mahmoud and Blue Larkspur, there are other large-heart lines that all trace to Eclipse. Papyrus, the source of Princequillo's heart, is also found in Favorite Trick, via Medieval Man through Honeyway. Ribot, Star Kingdom and Forli also pass on Papyrus's heart.

The great Double Jay heart that was found in John Henry and the Quarter Horse champion Sgt. Pepper Feature is also found in Mari's Book, who passed it on to Congaree, winner of the $500,000 Wood Memorial (G1) in 2001.

Man 'o War's heart is still racing today through horses from lines like Peaks and Valleys, Sandpit, Green Dancer, Hempen and Spy Song, among others. Damascus has given his heart to Dixieland Heat, Coronado's Quest, Ghazi, Red Ransom, Shadeed, Marlin and other progeny.

Domino, the source of the War Admiral heart through Sweep, is also passed through Stalwart. We measured a filly, Political Favor, last year, who may have one of the largest hearts we have ever found. The only source in her pedigree for a heart that size was Domino through Stalwart.

Stage Door Johnny passed an extraordinary heart to his daughters. We measured a daughter of his at Payson Stud last year and she had a 147-150 heart score. Another one of his daughters, Never Knock, has passed his heart to her sons Pleasant Tap and Go For Gin.

The stallion Storm Boot has been measured and passes Round Table's heart via Drumtop, with a heart score of 147. That extraordinary heart helps explain why he has sired such great daughters as graded stakes winners Bourbon Belle and Hurricane Bertie.

Alibhai was found to have a 14-pound heart at autopsy. He has proven to be a great broodmare sire, sending his heart down countless pedigrees through his daughters.

St. Simon, one of the most important sires in Thoroughbred history, has sent Eclipse's heart via Pocahontas into practically every pedigree of note in the past 100 years.

Native Dancer, who achieved immortality as the broodmare sire of Northern Dancer, is still a potent force in today's pedigrees. I believe that his heart is passed by Louis Quatorze, among others.

When it comes to passing great heart in today's pedigrees, War Admiral appears to have the edge. We know that it is a very large heart with great amplitude as well as a large heart score, and also seems to combine a tenacity and unwillingness to be headed that has brought great success to his descendants.

Following are some lists of horses that possibly carry specific heartlines. This is not a complete list as I haven't the space or time to find every horse ever bred that might carry particular lines. Instead, I have attempted to give a broad range of contemporary sires carrying important lines. There are many other horses carrying large hearts that trace back to to Eclipse in other ways that are not included, such as horses I've discussed earlier.

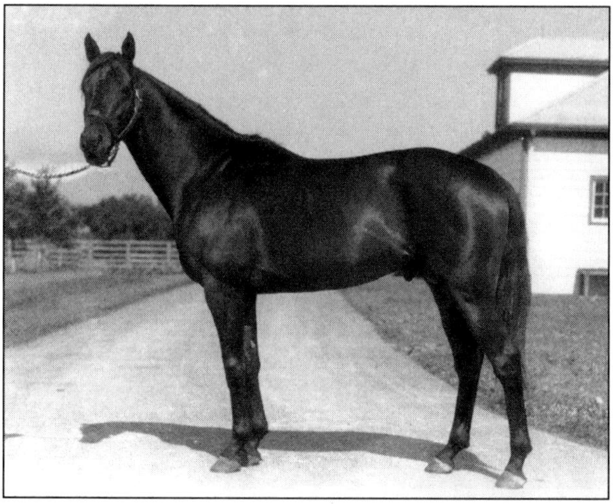

Photo courtesy of The Thoroughbred Times

War Admiral Heartline Stallions

Acceptable
Academy Award
Affirmed
Allen's Prospect
Alphabet Soup
Alysheba
American Chance
Behrens
Believe It
Better Self
Broad Brush
Bupers
Buckpasser
Cape Canaveral
Cape Town
Cherokee Run
Chester House
Crafty Admiral
Cryptoclearance
Cure The Blues
Deerhound
Desert Secret
Dr. Fager
Dubai Millennium
Easy Goer
El Gran Senor
Evansville Slew
Fappiano
Fast Play
Golden Missile
Great Above
Hoist The Flag
Housebuster
Irish Open
Judge TC
Keys to the Kingdom
Lear Fan
Lemon Drop Kid
Lomond
Miner's Mark
Mining
Mutakddin
Our Emblem
Personal Flag
Plugged Nickle
Polish Navy
Polish Numbers
Private Account
Quiet American
Rare Performer
Real Quiet
Roar
Romanov
Seattle Slew
Seeking The Gold
Silver Charm
Slew O' Gold
Stephanotis
Stormin Fever
Stormy Atlantic
Swaps
Top Account
Torrential
Touch Gold
Truckee
Wavering Monarch
Wild Rush
Will's Way
Woodman

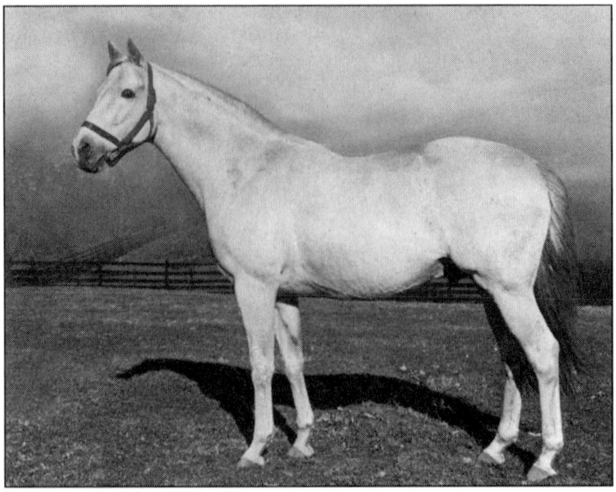

Photo courtesy of *The Thoroughbred Times*

Mahmoud Heartline Stallions

Arazi
Bucksplasher
Demon's Begone
El Prado
Flying Continental
Fusiachi Pegasus
Gallant Man
Gilded Time
Graustark
Halo
Harlan
His Majesty
Homebuilder
Lord Avie
Machiavellian
Majestic Prince
Mickey McGuire
Northern Dancer
Pine Bluff
Rahy
Rainbows For Life
Skip Trial
Silver Deputy
Silver Ghost
Southern Halo
Spectacular Bid
State Dinner
Tasso
Tossofthecoin
Waquoit
What A Pleasure
Wild Again
With Approval

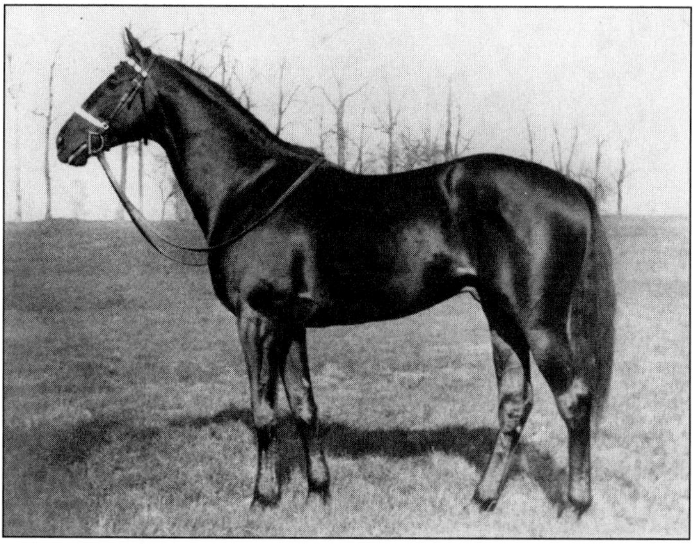

Photo courtesy of the Grayson/Sutcliffe Collection

Blue Larkspur Heartline Stallions

Alleged
Alydar
Alydeed
Bahri
Banker's Gold
Bates Motel
Batonnier
Big Spruce
Blushing John
Boldnesian
Bold Reason
Cat Thief
Caveat
Cohoes
Cozzene
Damascus
Dayjur
Devil's Bag
Fly So Free
General Meeting
Grey Dawn II
Holy Bull
Little Missouri
Lure
Never Bend
Nijinsky II
Opening Verse
Personal Hope
Prince John
Red Ransom
Relaunch
Riverman
Roberto
Saint Ballado
Scatmandu
Seattle Song
Skywalker
Slewpy
Smile
Stalwart
Subordination
Tiznow
TV Lark
Two Punch
Victory Speech
Wagon Limit
Zanthe

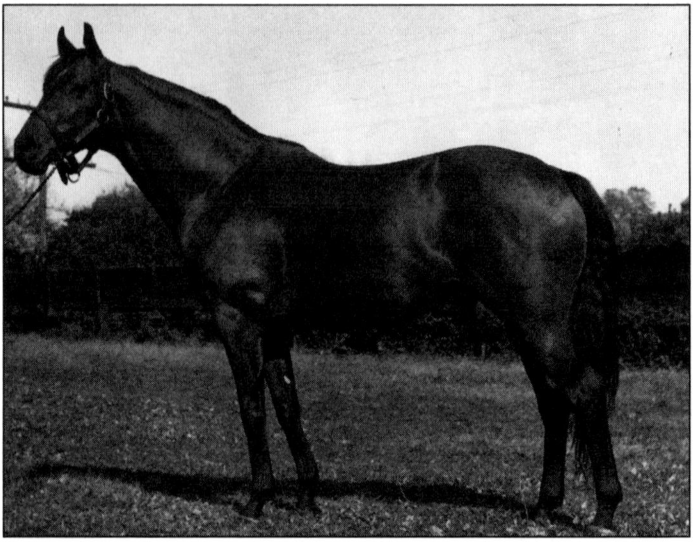

Photo courtesy of Keeneland Library/J.C. Skeets Meadors

Princequillo Heartline Stallions

Ack Ack
Afleet
Al Mamoon
A.P. Indy
Becker
Bold Bidder
Boone's Mill
Chief's Crown
Corporate Report
Danzig Connection
Diplomat Way
Dixie Brass
Dr. Blum
Farma Way
Galileo
Gone West
Grand Slam
Honor Grades
Indian Charlie
Key Contender
Key to the Mint
Kris S
Lion Cavern
Mill Reef
Miswaki
Moscow Ballet
Mountain Cat
One For All
Party Manners
Pleasant Colony
Quack
Roben Des Pins
Sham
Sir Gaylord
Skip Away
Smart Strike
Somethingfabulous
Succesor
Summer Squall
Swain
Sword Dance
Tiger Ridge
Vicar
Western Fame
Western Symphony
Yarrow Brae

Chapter 10

War Admiral

Of the four major super hearts in today's pedigrees, War Admiral is probably the most successful. His great heart, which came to him through his broodmare sire Sweep, who probably inherited it from the legendary Domino, has fueled countless racehorses, including three Triple Crown winners — War Admiral himself, Affirmed and Seattle Slew.

If you count the source, Sweep, then there are four Triple Crown winners including Whirlaway who, like War Admiral, was out of a daughter of Sweep.

In recent times there were two near misses — Silver Charm and Real Quiet. Both horses raced on War Admiral's heart. And the storied Cigar, who tied Citation's great record of 16 races in a row, also ran on the War Admiral heart.

The War Admiral X sent down through generations not only carries a great heart but a nearly unbeatable tenacity. Horses expressing this X don't like to be headed, and they will break themselves rather than surrender.

In addition to a large heart and racing tenacity, War Admiral had a high level of energy. He was elegant, racy and high-strung. Tom Harbut, 81, son of Man 'o War's famous groom Will Harbut, recalls exercising War Admiral.

He compared him with the antics of 2001 Preakness and Belmont Stakes winner Point Given who frequently went airborne, occasionally losing his rider while on the Triple Crown trail.

"Every time you got on War Admiral he would give three huge jumps," said Harbut. "You always had to remember there would be a third jump or you were in trouble. You didn't relax until he did all three. Then he was fine."

Harbut grew up around War Admiral's sire Man 'o War and said he will always regret not riding Man 'o War when he had the chance. "My brother exercised him and I rode War Admiral," he said. "We didn't think anything about it at the time. It was all part of our job and we were busy. But now, thinking back on it, I wish I had gotten on him just once so I could say I did."

There are those who have said that Man 'o War carried the fiery temperament attributed to his sire Fair Play. But according to Harbut, the only time Man 'o War was hard to handle was in the breeding shed. "There he was very aggressive," Harbut said. "But otherwise he wasn't hard to handle. He was very intelligent."

Harbut said War Admiral wasn't a big horse at 15.2-1/2 hands but was refined and full of fire. "He had plenty of heart."

War Admiral is an example of the size of a colt coming from the dam instead of the sire. In size he was unlike his strapping big sire, that stood at 16.2. He was built more like his broodmare sire Sweep. He was elegant and refined with a beautifully shaped head featuring medium-sized sculptured ears, large eyes, plenty of space in-between his jaws and a fine muzzle with oversized nostrils. He also had prominent withers with a beautifully sloped shoulder, long forearms and short cannons.

His aristocratic head with its small muzzle and large nostrils and wide space between his jaws is seen in his descendants expressing his X chromosome. If you compare the heads — especially from the front — of Escena, Lemon Drop Kid, Tale of Two Hearts, Desert Secret, Affirmed, Surfside, Seattle Slew, Silver Charm and Cigar, among others, you will see a striking family resemblance in the shape and expression of the head and face. The eyes are similarly set and can more easily see down the lane.

Because of the fire in him, War Admiral wasn't easy to keep weight on, something that has been handed down to his descendants. His head and front end are seen today in Broad Brush, Silver Charm, Lemon Drop Kid, Escena, Seattle Slew, Cigar and Seattle Slew daughters like Surfside, Desert Secret and Tale of Two

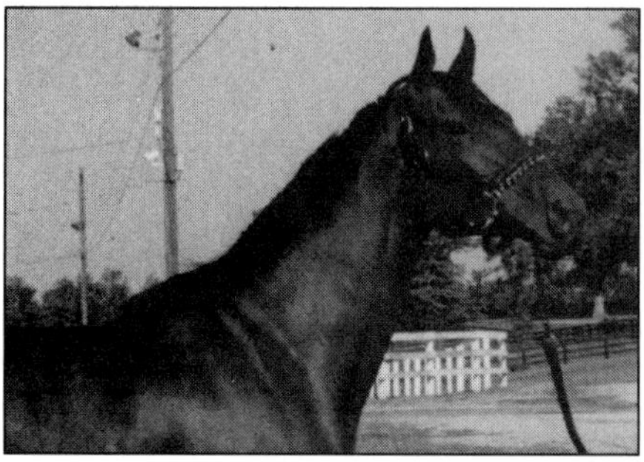

Tale of Two Hearts

Photo courtesy of Marianna Haun

Affirmed

Photo courtesy of Marianna Haun

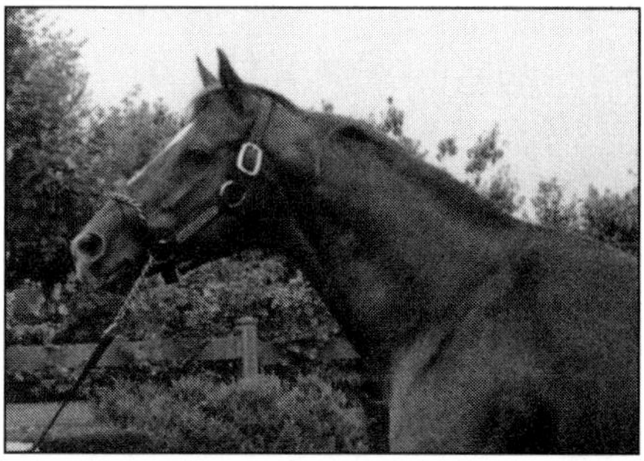

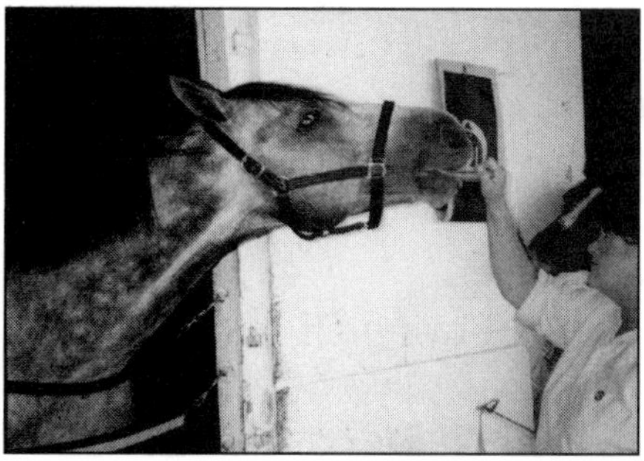

Silver Charm

Photo courtesy of Kellye Pikul

Desert Secret

Photo courtesy of Tony Leonard

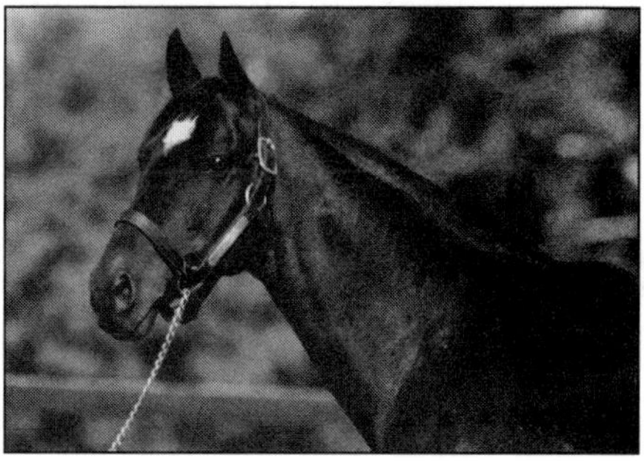

Hearts, to name a few. Wherever there is an expression of the War Admiral heart and X you will find physical similarities to his conformation, particularly in the head, top line and front end. Some are taller, but many are right around 15.3 to16 hands.

It is said of War Admiral that he traveled more like Sweep than Man 'o War. This makes sense if you consider the front end seems to follow the X expressed. In the War Admiral expression, there is an unusual way of going on the front end with the front leg rising higher from the forearm than is usually seen. This is a natural way of traveling for this line, but trainers are always trying to "level off" this way of going by the use of blinkers and shadow rolls. Sometimes this helps, but most often it doesn't change this peculiar way of traveling. Besides, as successful as this line has become there is really no need to worry about it.

War Admiral is his sire's most famous son. He is an example of what can happen when you take a great horse like Man 'o War and breed him to a mare with a heart even larger than his. With a heart score of 147-150, the War Admiral heart is larger than Man 'o War's, which was closer to 140.

War Admiral made 26 starts and won 21, with three seconds and one third, earning $273,240. He was only unplaced in one start. At three, he was unbeaten in eight starts, winning the Triple Crown and setting a new track record of 2:28 3/5 in the 11/2 mile Belmont Stakes, which equaled the American record.

His sire Man 'o War had won 20 of his 21 starts, earning $249,465. He set world records at 1 3/8 miles and 1 5/8 miles, track records at 1 1/4 miles and in the Belmont Stakes at 1 1/2 miles, the same stakes his son would later break the track record in as well.

The brilliantly fast Dr. Fager carried the War Admiral heart; he didn't like to give in either. Damascus was only able to beat him twice, once when Damascus's trainer sent out a world-record holding rabbit in Hedavar. Dr. Fager could not stand to let him get away and burned himself out trying to beat Hedavar, allowing Damascus to get past him at the end. Dr. Fager had amazing speed, holding a world record for the mile for more than 30 years, but he didn't have patience, just great heart.

In the stirring battles between Affirmed and Alydar, both horses had hearts of similar great size, but Affirmed had that tenacity that comes with the War Admiral heart and he wouldn't let Alydar pass him.

Affirmed passed speed and heart to his offspring, siring Canadian champion Peteski, winner of more than $1.2 million, and two-time champion Flawlessly, winner of more than $2.5 million.

Seattle Slew was the only undefeated Triple Crown winner. He sent his great heart to his daughters which passed it on to their offspring like Cigar, who held off his competitors for a record 16 races in a row.

Broad Brush, who carries the War Admiral heart, won more than $2.6 million while winning such prestigious races as the Wood Memorial (G1), the Santa Anita Handicap (G1), the Meadowlands Cup Handicap (G1) and the Suburban Handicap (G1). He has become a very successful sire, siring both top sons and daughters including his son Concern, winner of the Breeders' Cup Classic (G1).

Fappiano, who carried the War Admiral heart of his dam Killaloe, a daughter of Dr. Fager, has proven to be a tremendous sire even though he only had nine crops before his death. He passed his speed to his sons and his heart to his daughters. Among his sons are champion Unbridled, who is inbred to War Admiral, both top and bottom; champion Rubiano; champion Tasso; Cryptoclearance, winner of more than $3.3million; and Quiet American, sire of Kentucky Derby winner Real Quiet. Among his daughters is Tappiano, G1 winner of more than $1.3 million. Fappiano daughters have become sought after as great producers.

Buckpasser was a superb example of what the War Admiral heart could do, both on the track and in the breeding shed. Daughters of Buckpasser became like drops of gold when it came to producing racehorses. When Buckpasser daughters met Mr. Prospector with his blazing speed, the sons that were produced became legendary.

One Buckpasser grandson was Seeking the Gold out of Con Game by Buckpasser. Seeking the Gold earned more than

$2.3 million and sired such daughters as champion Heavenly Prize, champion Flanders, and Seeking the Pearl, winner of more than $4 million. When bred to large-hearted mares he sired sons like Cape Town out of a Seattle Slew mare, that also carried the War Admiral heart, and G1-winner Dubai Millennium, winner of the Dubai

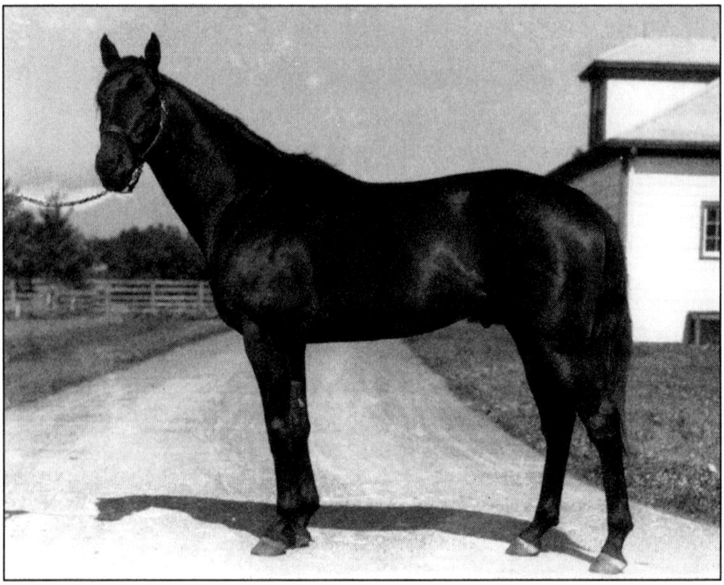

Photo courtesy of the Thoroughbred Times

War Admiral

World Cup. Seeking the Gold sons and daughters draw high bids at the major sales, and rightly so.

Among War Admiral's greatest daughters were Bee Mac, who won the Spinaway and Hopeful Stakes, the great champion Busher who was Horse of the Year in 1945 just like her sire was in 1937, and Striking, Busher's full-sister. Striking would become the better producer, passing on her sire's heart to Triple Crown winner Seattle Slew through My Charmer, daughter of Poker, and to Kentucky Derby winner Silver Charm via another Poker daughter, Bonnie's Poker.

Cigar and Bonnie's Poker were measured and had the same

War Admiral
1934

- Man 'o War
  - Fair Play
    - Hastings
      - Spendthrift
        - Australian
        - Aerolite
      - Cinderella
        - Tomahawk
        - Manna
    - Fairy Gold
      - Bend Or
        - Doncaster
        - Rouge Rose
      - Dame Masham
        - Galliard
        - Pauline
  - Mahubah
    - Rock Sand
      - Sainfoin
        - Springfield
        - Sanda
      - Roquebrune
        - St. Simon
        - St. Marguerite
    - Merry Token
      - Merry Hampton
        - Hampton
        - Doll Tearsheet
      - Mizpah
        - Macgregor
        - Mare by Underhand
- Brushup
  - Sweep
    - Ben Brush
      - Bramble
        - Bonnie Scotland
        - Ivy Leaf
      - Roseville
        - Reform
        - Albia
    - Pink Domino
      - Domino
        - Himayar
        - Mannie Gray
      - Bell Rose
        - Beaudesert
        - MonteRose
  - Annette K.
    - Harry of Hereford
      - John 'o Gaunt
        - Isinglass
        - La Fleche
      - Canterbury Pilgrim
        - Tristan
        - Pilgrimage
    - Bathing Girl
      - Spearmint
        - Carbine
        - Maid of the Mint
      - Summer Girl
        - Sundridge
        - Permission

heart score. Tale of Two Hearts, who was bred to have the My Charmer heart, also had the same heart score of 147-150. Their ECG tracings were similar as well with a wide base and very high amplitude. We don't know why but some of the greatest hearts combine high heart score with high amplitude.

When you compare the ECG tracings of Cigar, Alysheba, Desert Secret, Fappiano daughters, Bonnie's Poker, Tale of Two Hearts, Desert Secret, Huddle Up, Private Account, El Gran Senor and Woodman, all of whom express the War Admiral heart, there is a definite family resemblance not only in terms of heart score, but in terms of the QRS wave and high amplitude found in these tracings.

This is something new. We knew that the heart scores of particular hearts were very consistent. But until we started compiling and comparing the various heartlines via their ECGs we didn't realize how strong the resemblance was between hearts that came from many different directions all carrying the same specific heart, such as the War Admiral heart.

The same thing was seen in other family groupings such as Key to the Mint and his daughters and descendants. Moscow Ballet and his daughters also shared a similar tracing and heart score.

Northern Sunset, the foundation mare at Payson Stud who passes the Northfields heart, gave the same size and tracing to three of her sons that we measured: St. Jovite, Salem Drive, and Lac Ouimet. In terms of physical clues to genetic traits, it was interesting to note that Northern Sunset shared a strong resemblance with Spinning World, whose second dam was by Northfields. From this observation, it is possible to speculate that Spinning World probably shares her 140 heart score.

There is still much to learn about the genetic trail along the X line. But the recurring patterns of specific traits in addition to specific hearts following certain Xs is hard to ignore.

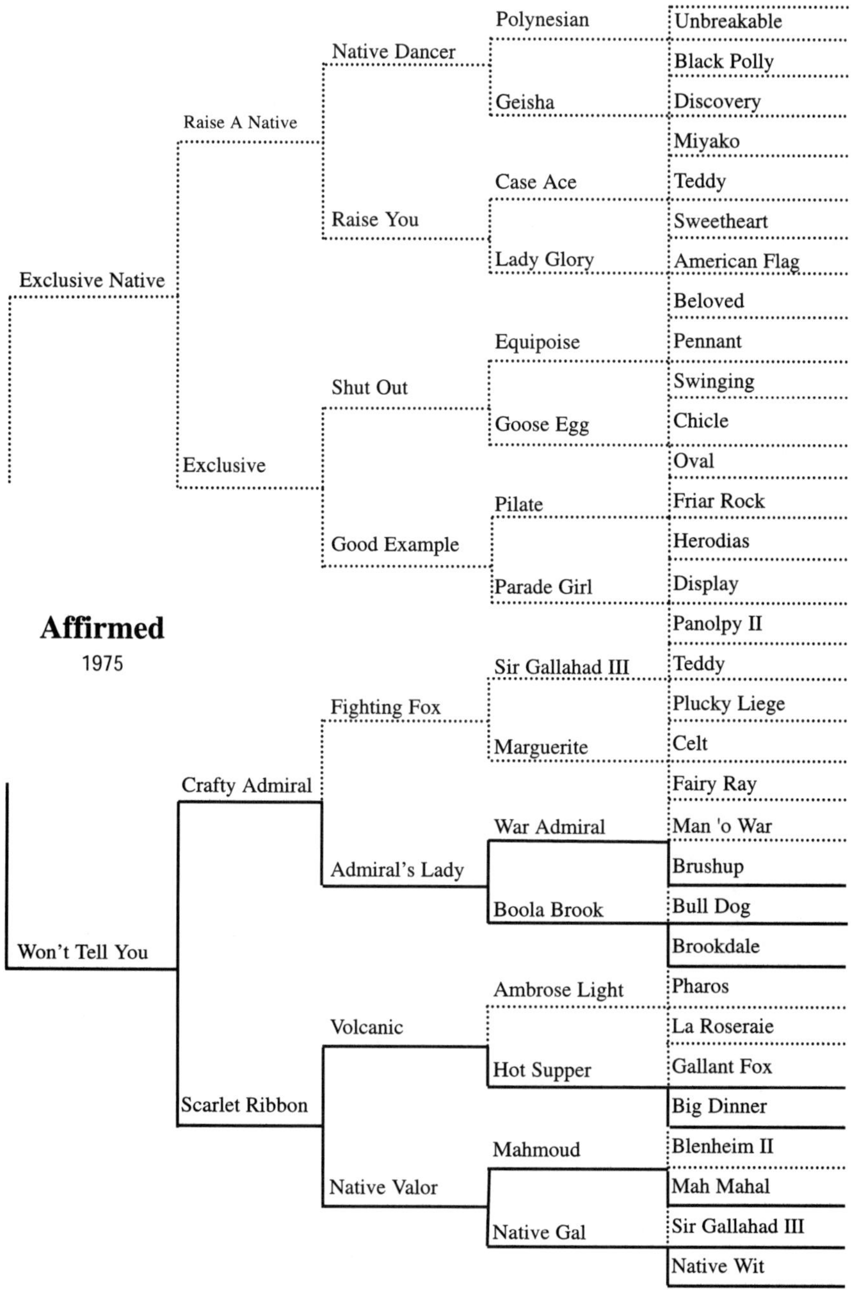
Affirmed
1975
Exclusive Native
Raise A Native
Native Dancer
Polynesian
Unbreakable
Black Polly
Geisha
Discovery
Miyako
Raise You
Case Ace
Teddy
Sweetheart
Lady Glory
American Flag
Beloved
Exclusive
Shut Out
Equipoise
Pennant
Swinging
Goose Egg
Chicle
Oval
Good Example
Pilate
Friar Rock
Herodias
Parade Girl
Display
Panolpy II
Won't Tell You
Crafty Admiral
Fighting Fox
Sir Gallahad III
Teddy
Plucky Liege
Marguerite
Celt
Fairy Ray
Admiral's Lady
War Admiral
Man 'o War
Brushup
Boola Brook
Bull Dog
Brookdale
Scarlet Ribbon
Volcanic
Ambrose Light
Pharos
La Roseraie
Hot Supper
Gallant Fox
Big Dinner
Native Valor
Mahmoud
Blenheim II
Mah Mahal
Native Gal
Sir Gallahad III
Native Wit

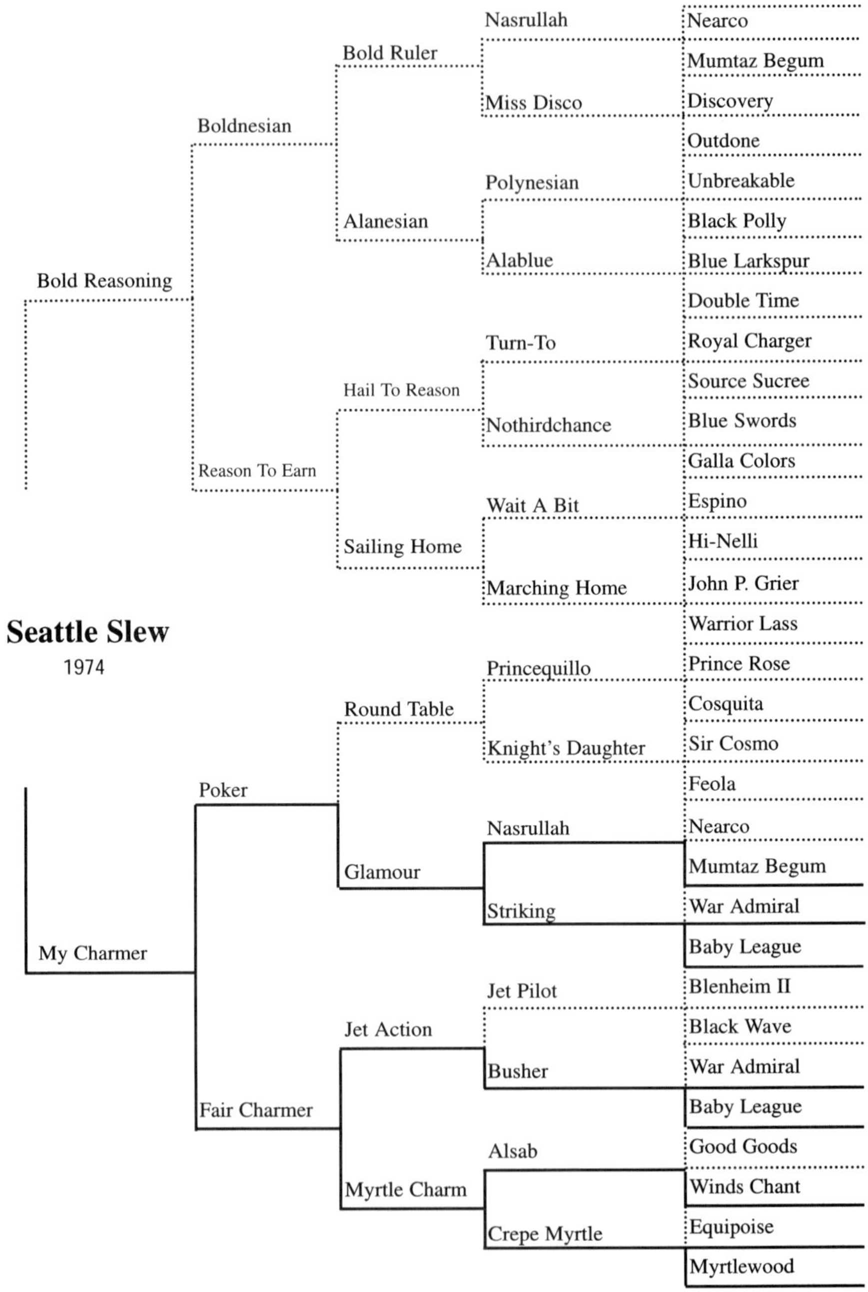
Seattle Slew
1974
Bold Reasoning
Boldnesian
Bold Ruler
Nasrullah
Nearco
Mumtaz Begum
Miss Disco
Discovery
Outdone
Alanesian
Polynesian
Unbreakable
Black Polly
Alablue
Blue Larkspur
Double Time
Reason To Earn
Hail To Reason
Turn-To
Royal Charger
Source Sucree
Nothirdchance
Blue Swords
Galla Colors
Sailing Home
Wait A Bit
Espino
Hi-Nelli
Marching Home
John P. Grier
Warrior Lass
My Charmer
Poker
Round Table
Princequillo
Prince Rose
Cosquita
Knight's Daughter
Sir Cosmo
Feola
Glamour
Nasrullah
Nearco
Mumtaz Begum
Striking
War Admiral
Baby League
Fair Charmer
Jet Action
Jet Pilot
Blenheim II
Black Wave
Busher
War Admiral
Baby League
Myrtle Charm
Alsab
Good Goods
Winds Chant
Crepe Myrtle
Equipoise
Myrtlewood

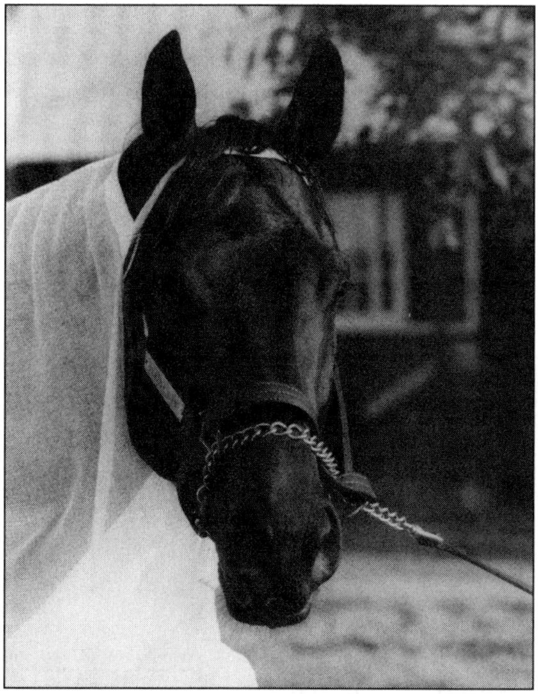

Photo courtesy of ***the Thoroughbred Times***

Seattle Slew
(Bold Reasoning x My Charmer)

Broad Brush

1983

Parents	Grandparents	Great-grandparents	3rd generation	4th generation
Ack Ack	Battle Joined	Armageddon	Alsab	Good Goods
				Winds Chant
			Fighting Lady	Sir Gallahad III
				Lady Nicotine
		Ethel Walker	Revoked	Blue Larkspur
				Gala Belle
			Ethel Terry	Reaping Reward
				Mary Terry
	Fast Turn	Turn-To	Royal Charger	Nearco
				Sun Princess
			Source Sucree	Admiral Drake
				Lavendula II
		Cherokee Rose	Princequillo	Prince Rose
				Cosquillo
			The Squaw II	Sickle
				Minnewaska
Hay Patcher	Hoist The Flag	Tom Rolfe	Ribot	Tenerani
				Romanella
			Pocahontas	Roman
				How
		Wavy Navy	War Admiral	Man 'o War
				Brushup
			Triomphe	Tourbillon
				Melibee
	Turn To Talent	Turn-To	Royal Charger	Nearco
				Sun Princess
			Source Sucree	Admiral Drake
				Lavendula II
		Hidden Talent	Dark Star	Royal Gem II
				Isolde
			Dangerous Dame	Nasrullah
				Lady Kells

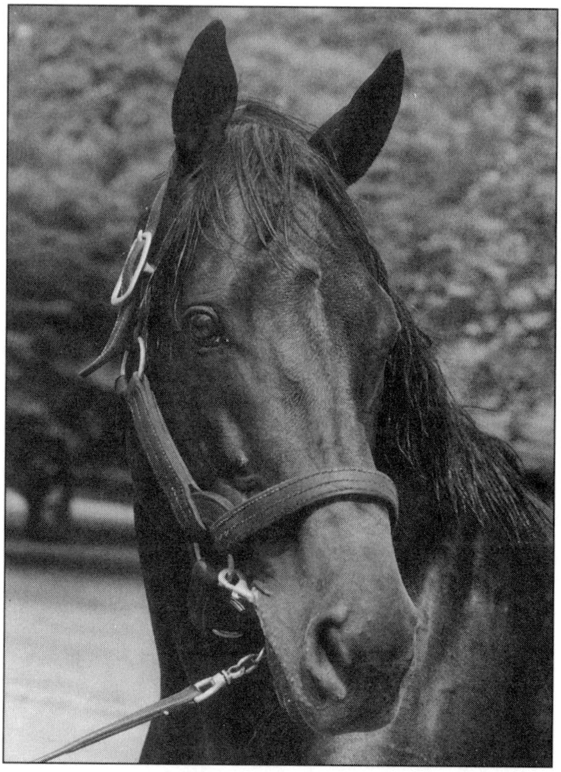

Photo courtesy of Marianna Haun

Broad Brush
(Ack Ack x Hay Patcher)

Lemon Drop Kid

1996

- Kingmambo
  - Mr. Prospector
    - Raise A Native
      - Native Dancer
        - Polynesian
        - Geisha
      - Raise You
        - Case Ace
        - Lady Glory
    - Gold Digger
      - Nashua
        - Nasrullah
        - Segula
      - Sequence
        - Count Fleet
        - Miss Dogwood
  - Miesque
    - Nureyev
      - Northern Dancer
        - Nearctic
        - Natalma
      - Special
        - Forli
        - Thong
    - Pasadoble
      - Prove Out
        - Graustark
        - Equal Venture
      - Santa Quilla
        - Sanctus
        - Neriad
- Charming Lassie
  - Seattle Slew
    - Bold Reasoning
      - Boldnesian
        - Bold Ruler
        - Alanesian
      - Reason To Earn
        - Hail to Reason
        - Sailing Home
    - My Charmer
      - Poker
        - Round Table
        - Glamour
      - Fair Charmer
        - Jet Action
        - Myrtle Charm
  - Lassie Dear
    - Buckpasser
      - Tom Fool
        - Menow
        - Gaga
      - Busanda
        - War Admiral
        - Businesslike
    - Gay Missle
      - Sir Gaylord
        - Turn-To
        - Somethingroyal
      - Missy Baba
        - My Babu
        - Ulvira II

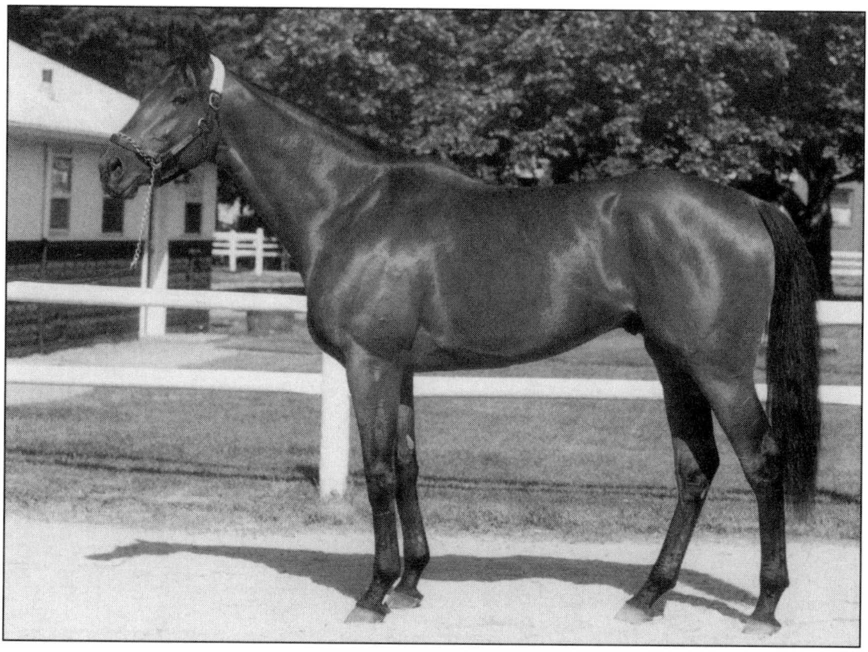

Photo courtesy of the Thoroughbred Times

Lemon Drop Kid
(Kingmambo x Charming Lassie)

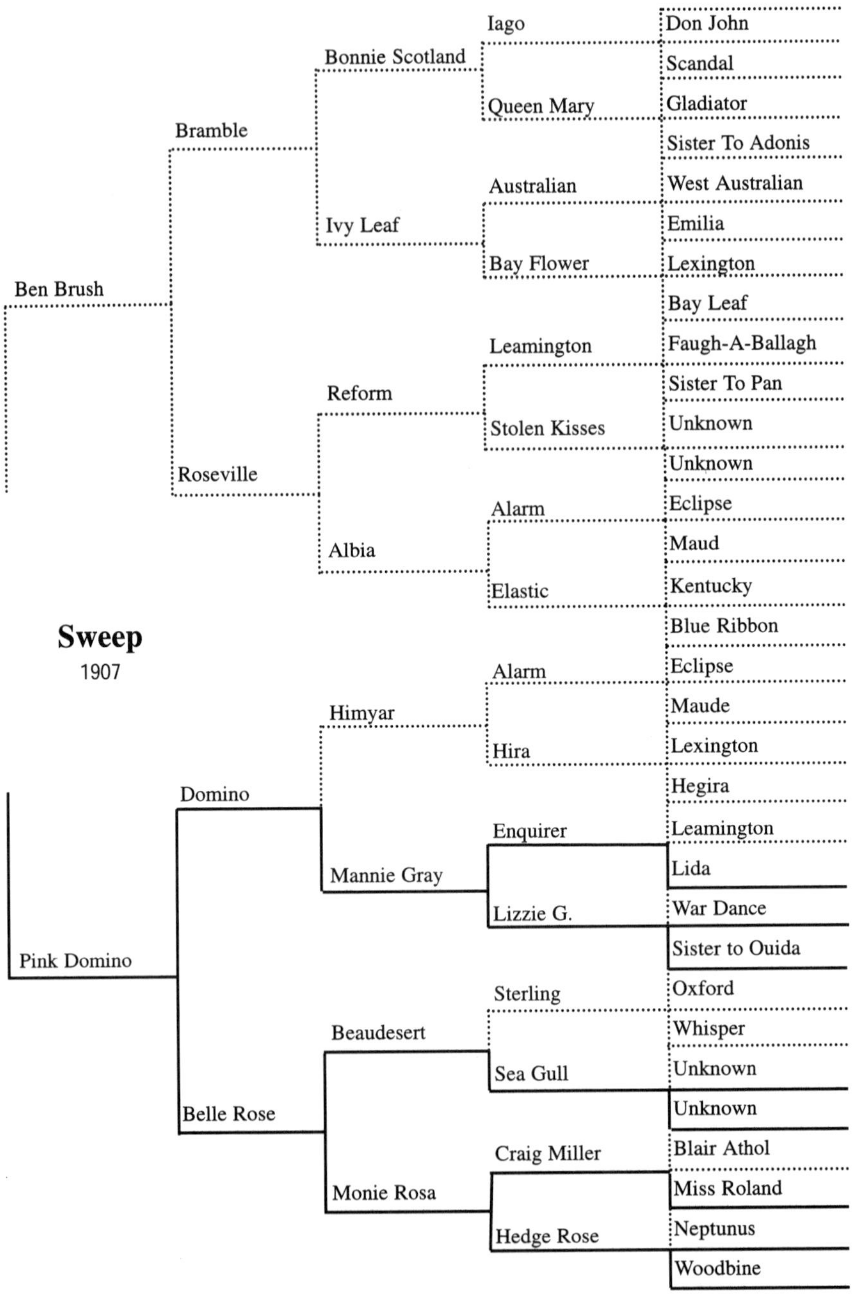
Sweep
1907
Ben Brush
Bramble
Bonnie Scotland
Iago
Don John
Scandal
Queen Mary
Gladiator
Sister To Adonis
Ivy Leaf
Australian
West Australian
Emilia
Bay Flower
Lexington
Bay Leaf
Roseville
Reform
Leamington
Faugh-A-Ballagh
Sister To Pan
Stolen Kisses
Unknown
Unknown
Albia
Alarm
Eclipse
Maud
Elastic
Kentucky
Blue Ribbon
Pink Domino
Domino
Himyar
Alarm
Eclipse
Maude
Hira
Lexington
Hegira
Mannie Gray
Enquirer
Leamington
Lida
Lizzie G.
War Dance
Sister to Ouida
Belle Rose
Beaudesert
Sterling
Oxford
Whisper
Sea Gull
Unknown
Unknown
Monie Rosa
Craig Miller
Blair Athol
Miss Roland
Hedge Rose
Neptunus
Woodbine

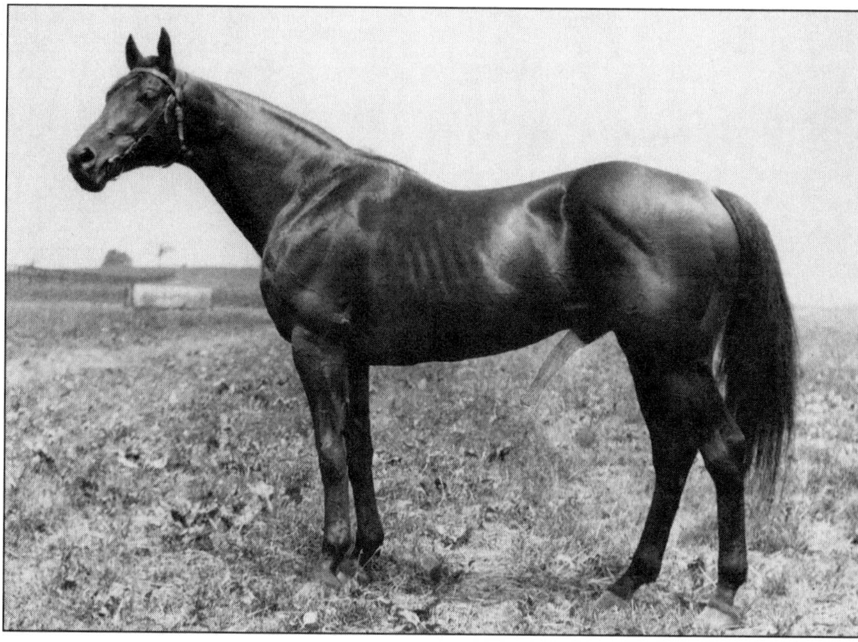

Photo courtesy of the Grayson/Sutcliffe Collection

Sweep (top) and Domino (bottom)

Photo courtesy of the Grayson/Sutcliffe Collection

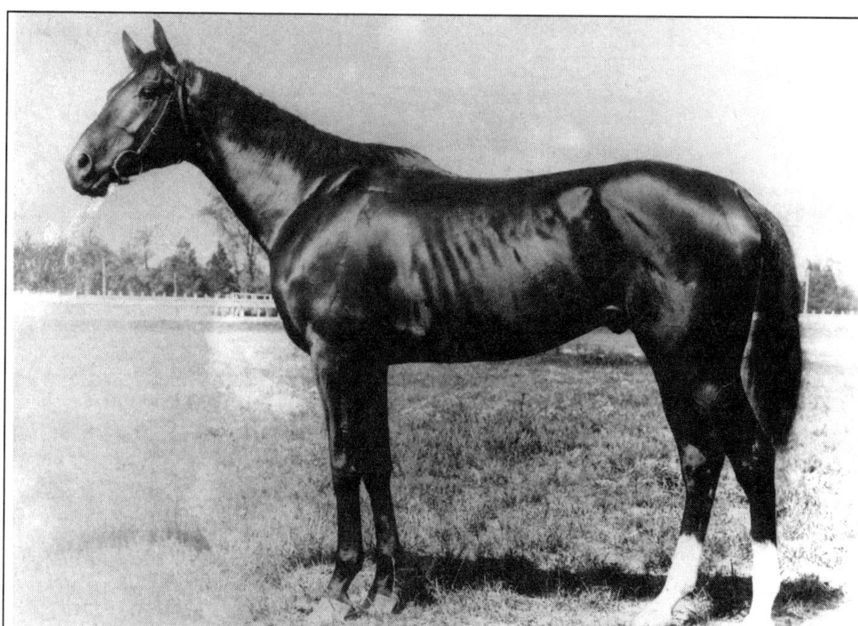

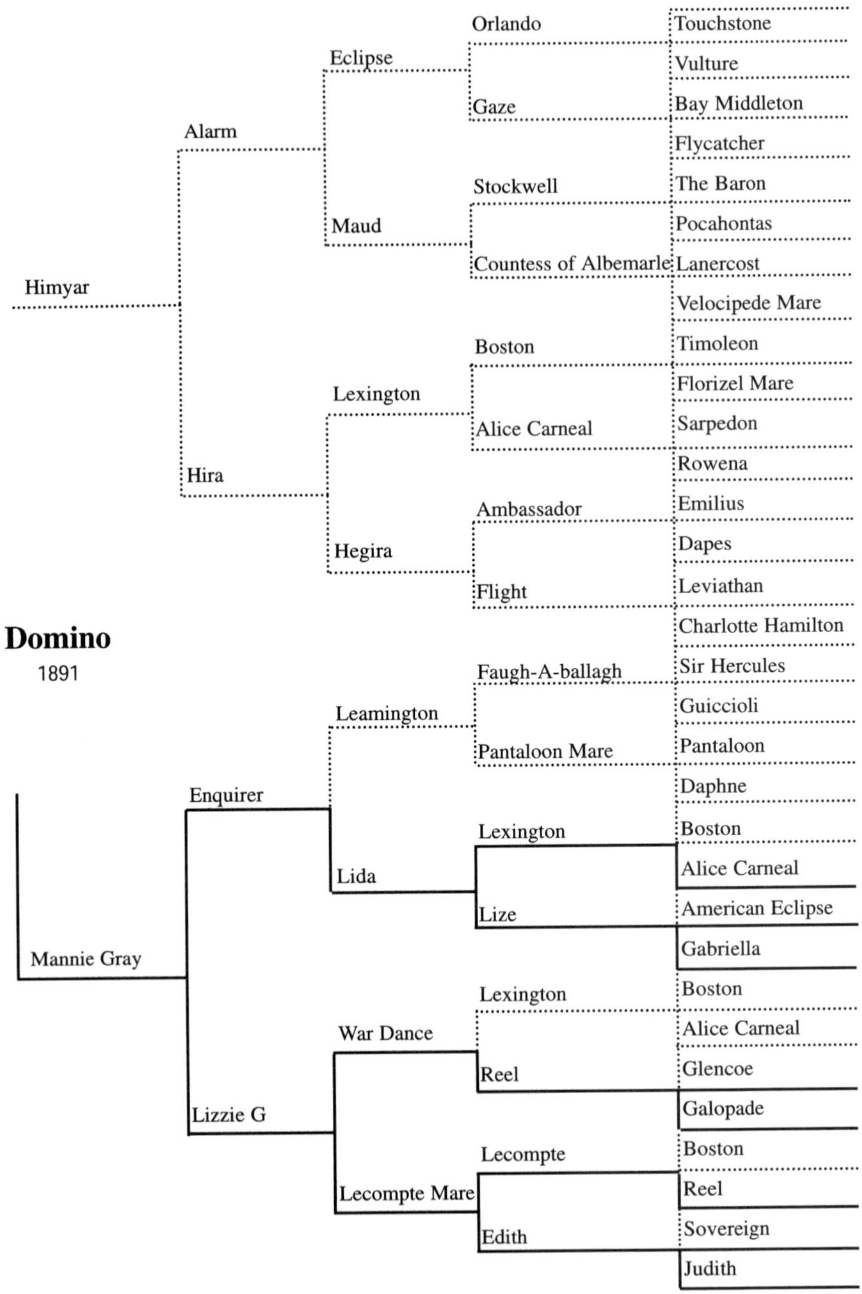
Domino
1891
Himyar
Alarm
Eclipse
Orlando
Touchstone
Vulture
Gaze
Bay Middleton
Flycatcher
Maud
Stockwell
The Baron
Pocahontas
Countess of Albemarle
Lanercost
Velocipede Mare
Hira
Lexington
Boston
Timoleon
Florizel Mare
Alice Carneal
Sarpedon
Rowena
Hegira
Ambassador
Emilius
Dapes
Flight
Leviathan
Charlotte Hamilton
Mannie Gray
Enquirer
Leamington
Faugh-A-ballagh
Sir Hercules
Guiccioli
Pantaloon Mare
Pantaloon
Daphne
Lida
Lexington
Boston
Alice Carneal
Lize
American Eclipse
Gabriella
Lizzie G
War Dance
Lexington
Boston
Alice Carneal
Reel
Glencoe
Galopade
Lecompte Mare
Lecompte
Boston
Reel
Edith
Sovereign
Judith

Chapter 11

Tiny Twin With a Big Heart

As part of our study of the X Factor, we bred the 14.2 twin mare The Last Red, a double-copy mare, to Alysheba. We had measured Alysheba and discovered that he carried the War Admiral heart from his second dam Belthazar, a daughter of War Admiral. Alysheba has a heart score of 147.

We decided on this breeding because Alysheba was a typical large-hearted champion who was panned as a sire because he couldn't reproduce himself in a son. Knowing that his great heart could only be given to a daughter, the solution seemed obvious. Take a mare, even a tiny twin, with a great heart as large as his to supply the engine for his son.

I was praying for a filly with Alysheba's heart, but the magnificent colt I got more than made up for my disappointment. The only question with the colt was which X The Last Red would give him.

We had already identified both sex-linked X chromosomes carried by The Last Red, both expressed and recessive. We had done this by measuring all the foals of her dam Sissy's Time, her sire Moscow Ballet, and her own foals.

On one, the dominant X that she expressed, The Last Red carried her sire's large Princequillo heart. On the other, she carried the recessive X of her broodmare sire,Villamor, a son of Native Dancer, who carried the X he inherited from his second dam Rampart, a daughter of Boat by Man 'o War.

Villamor's dam Dianthus was a daughter of Your Host, who

carried the Mahmoud heart inherited from his dam Boudoir II. Because of the very specific small round ears that follow the Mahmoud X, it was easy to determine that Villamor didn't inherit his heart from Your Host. But his physical characteristics did match up with Rampart and Man 'o War.

When Mighty Mouse, as The Last Red is nicknamed, produced a colt that looked nothing like his brother and very much like Man 'o War and Alydar, it was easy to figure out her recessive X. This was the X she gave to the colt she produced from the Alysheba mating. He inherited not only Man 'o War's heart, but his front end, carriage, ears and eyes.

The Alysheba colt's birth, on a tobacco farm outside of Paris, Ky., was one of the strangest I have ever witnessed. Because Mighty Mouse always foals early, it is hard to know exactly when she will foal. After spending several nights in the barn when it looked like she would foal at any moment, she finally started.We discovered the foal had his left leg bent back at the knee and we had to reach in and pull it forward.

The mare lay down and the foal started to come out. This is the strange part: He was only out just past his withers when he literally sat up. The sac fell off him and his head was lifted with his neck erect. (We would later realize that that neck and head carriage came from his famous ancestor, Man 'o War.) He was sniffing the air, curling his lip. He could smell the milk that Mighty Mouse had released and he started hollering his head off.

I couldn't believe it. He wasn't even all the way out into the world and he looked like a centaur sticking out of his mother, neighing and curling his upper lip. When we got him the rest of the way out, he was quickly up and amazingly coordinated.

Then he faced the same problem that all of Mighty Mouse's big babies face. They can't believe how far down the milk is and they keep poking her in the middle of her barrel, sure that there is a tap there somewhere. He was up for an hour before he was finally ready to lay down and take a nap.

All of Mighty Mouse's babies have been big and coordinated but nothing like this one. He was born with such attitude that we were joking in the barn that he seemed to be saying, "My daddy won the Kentucky Derby."

Mighty Mouse has produced four foals, two daughters and two sons. She was nice enough to give a different X to each of her sons. Her two daughters both expressed their sires' hearts. All four foals look nothing alike; they each have a different body type and a different large heart. All were above normal size.

While very small because she only weighed 52 pounds at birth and had only a 30 percent attachment to her placenta, Mighty Mouse produces very large foals. And she kicks them out early.

Her first foal, a filly by Desert Secret, that is now 15.2-1/2 hands (the exact size of War Admiral whose X she carries), was born three weeks early and weighed 110 pounds. She was fat, straight and very alert at birth. If it were not for the ultrasounds, you would have sworn you had the wrong conception date. This filly has been measured and has the same large heart as Seattle Slew, Silver Charm and Cigar, with a heart score of 147-150.

Mighty Mouse's second foal, a filly by Lake George, weighed 142 pounds and was about eight days early. She was on the way to a height of 16.2 when she lost her life in a tragic accident during training as a two-year-old.

Her third foal was her first colt. By Huddle Up, he weighed about 130 pounds and was about two weeks early. He looked like his dam and reached a height of 15.3, the size of his maternal grandsire Moscow Ballet. That was the heart he inherited and he has demonstrated great endurance during his training.

Height seems to follow the X chromosome that is expressed. For centuries, the Middle Eastern Arabian breeders have maintained that the mare determines the size of the foal. That is true, but that size depends upon which X that foal inherits. In the case of a filly, if she expresses her sire's X, then she should approach his height. With a colt, it depends upon which side of his mother's family he inherits. While the height seems to be pretty consistent, there does appear to be a "blending" on this characteristic. There are cases where the sire was very tall and the resulting foal is somewhere in between the size of the sire and dam.

The Huddle Up colt was the size of Moscow Ballet. The Alysheba colt, who at 14 months was already more than 15 hands tall, will be the same 16.2 as his broodmare sire Villamor, as well as Man 'o War.

In measuring more than 1,000 horses, we have noticed there are physical clues as to which X came up in the mix. Not only are the ears a genetic marker for specific hearts, but other family resemblances appear to follow the X that is expressed.

Because of his resemblance to his famous ancestor, the Alysheba colt was registered as Man 'o Sheba. He also bears a striking resemblance to his paternal grandsire Alydar. He is marked like Alydar and has his head, with Man 'o War's ears and eyes.

Another thing that was noticed with this colt was the muscle mass that seems to appear when Raise A Native and Native Dancer are inbred as they were in this particular mating. Northern Dancer was also inbred in this match. Pedigree experts often talk about the heavy muscle that seems to follow the inbreeding of Raise A Native/Northern Dancer/Native Dancer/Mr. Prospector. I don't believe that muscle mass is sex-linked, but it can be inbred.

While our project is specifically following the large-heart genetic mutation, it is impossible not to recognize other patterns of inheritance, especially in terms of family resemblance seen on the X line.

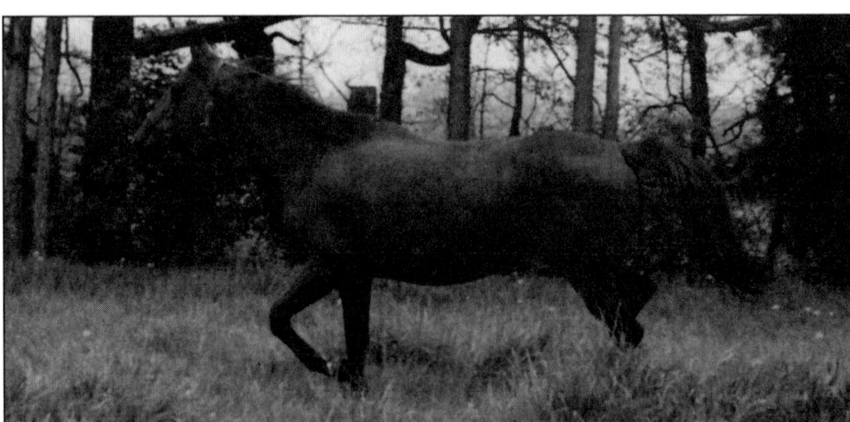

Photo courtesy of Marianna Haun

The Last Red (Moscow Ballet x Sissy's Time)

The Last Red
1993

- Moscow Ballet
  - Nijinsky II
    - Northern Dancer
      - Nearctic
        - Nearco
        - Lady Angela
      - Natalma
        - Native Dancer
        - Almahmoud
    - Flaming Page
      - Bull Page
        - Bull Lea
        - Our Page
      - Flaring Top
        - Menow
        - Flaming Top
  - Millicent
    - Cornish Prince
      - Bold Ruler
        - Nasrullah
        - Miss Disco
      - Teleran
        - Eight Thirty
        - Tellaris
    - Milan Mill
      - Princequillo
        - Prince Rose
        - Cosquilla
      - Virginia Water
        - Count Fleet
        - Red Ray
- Sissy's Time
  - Villamor
    - Native Dancer
      - Polynesian
        - Unbreakable
        - Black Polly
      - Geisha
        - Discovery
        - Miyako
    - Dianthus
      - Your Host
        - Alibhai
        - Boudoir II
      - Rampart
        - Trace Call
        - Boat
  - Page Book
    - Needles
      - Ponder
        - Pensive
        - Miss Rushin
      - Noodle Soup
        - Jack High
        - Supromene
    - Imprint
      - War Relic
        - Man 'o War
        - Friar's Carse
      - In The Purple
        - Burgoo King
        - Black Helen

Man 'o Sheba

2000

Parents	Grandparents	Great-grandparents	Great-great-grandparents	
Alysheba	Alydar	Raise A Native	Native Dancer	Polynesian
				Geisha
			Raise You	Case Ace
				Lady Glory
		Sweet Tooth	On-And-On	Nasrullah
				Two Lea
			Plum Cake	Ponder
				Real Delight
	Bel Sheba	Lt Stevens	Nantallah	Nasrullah
				Shimmer
			Rough Shod	Gold Bridge
				Dalmary
		Belthazar	War Admiral	Man 'o War
				Brushup
			Blinking Owl	Pharamond II
				Baba Kenny
The Last Red	Moscow Ballet	Nijinsky II	Northern Dancer	Nearctic
				Natalma
			Flaming Page	Bull Page
				Flaring Top
		Millicent	Cornish Prince	Bold Ruler
				Teleran
			Milan Mill	Princquillo
				Virginia Water
	Sissy's Time	Villamor	Native Dancer	Polynesian
				Geisha
			Dianthus	Your Host
				Rampart
		Page Book	Needles	Ponder
				Noodle Soup
			Imprint	War Relic
				In The Purple

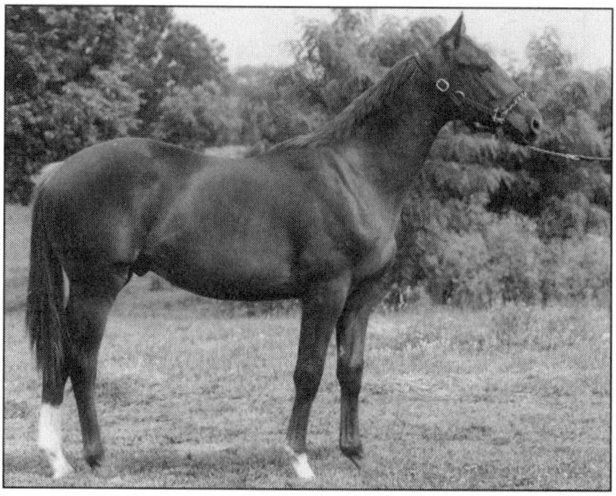

Man 'o Sheba
(Alysheba x
The Last Red)

Photo courtesy of Marianna Haun

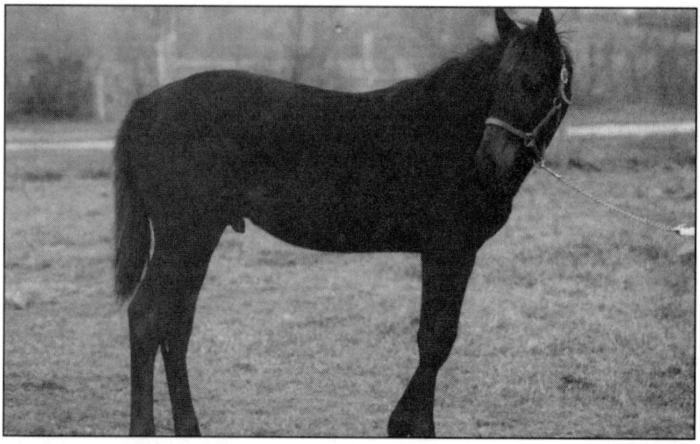

Heart of Jaws
(Huddle Up x
The Last Red)

Photo courtesy of Marianna Haun

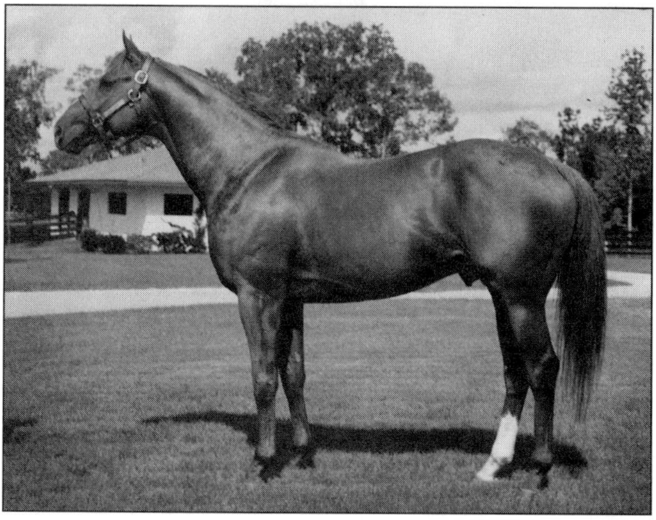

Villamor,
broodmare sire
of The Last Red
and son of
Native Dancer.

Photo courtesy of Jim Jernigan

Heart of Jaws

1999

- Huddle Up
  - Sir Ivor
    - Sir Gaylord
      - Turn-To
        - Royal Charger
        - Source Sucree
      - Somethingroyal
        - Princequillo
        - Imperatrice
    - Attica
      - Mr Trouble
        - Mahmoud
        - Motto
      - Athenia
        - Pharamond II
        - Salaminia
  - Huggle Duggle
    - Never Bend
      - Nasrullah
        - Nearco
        - Mumtaz Begum
      - Lalun
        - Djeddah
        - Be Faithful
    - Crown The Queen
      - Swaps
        - Khaled
        - Iron Reward
      - Village Beauty
        - My Babu
        - Spring Tune
- The Last Red
  - Moscow Ballet
    - Nijinsky II
      - Northern Dancer
        - Nearctic
        - Natalma
      - Flaming Page
        - Bull Page
        - Flaring Top
    - Millicent
      - Cornish Prince
        - Bold Ruler
        - Teleran
      - Milan Mill
        - Princequillo
        - Virginia Water
  - Sissy's Time
    - Villamor
      - Native Dancer
        - Polynesian
        - Geisha
      - Dianthus
        - Your Host
        - Rampart
    - Page Book
      - Needles
        - Ponder
        - Noodle Soup
      - Imprint
        - War Relic
        - In The Purple

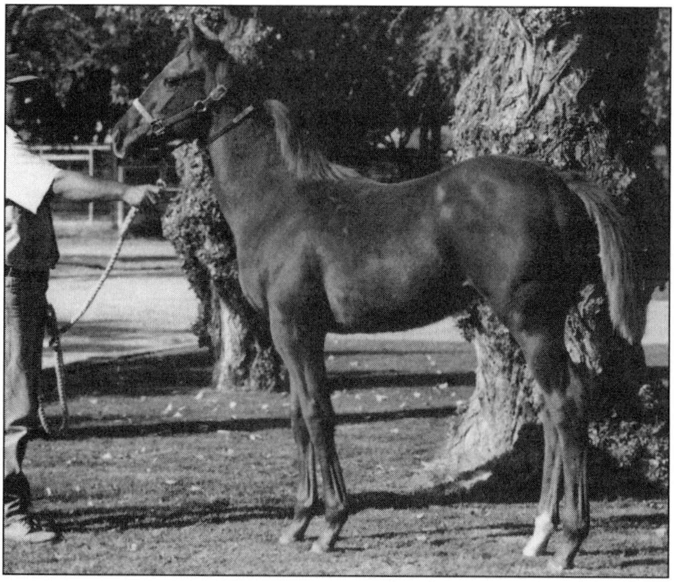

Heartmaker
(Lake George
x The Last Red)

Photo courtesy of Marianna Haun

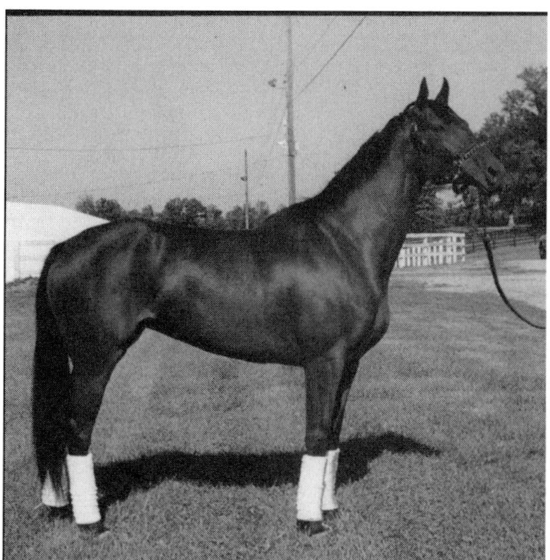

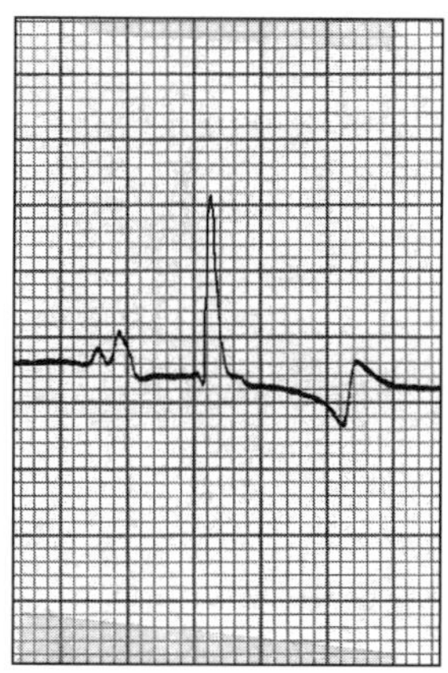

Photo courtesy of Marianna Haun; ECG courtesy of Dr. Fred Fregin

Tale of Two Hearts, out of The Last Red by Desert Secret, and her ECG.
Her heart score was measured at 147.

Heartmaker

1998

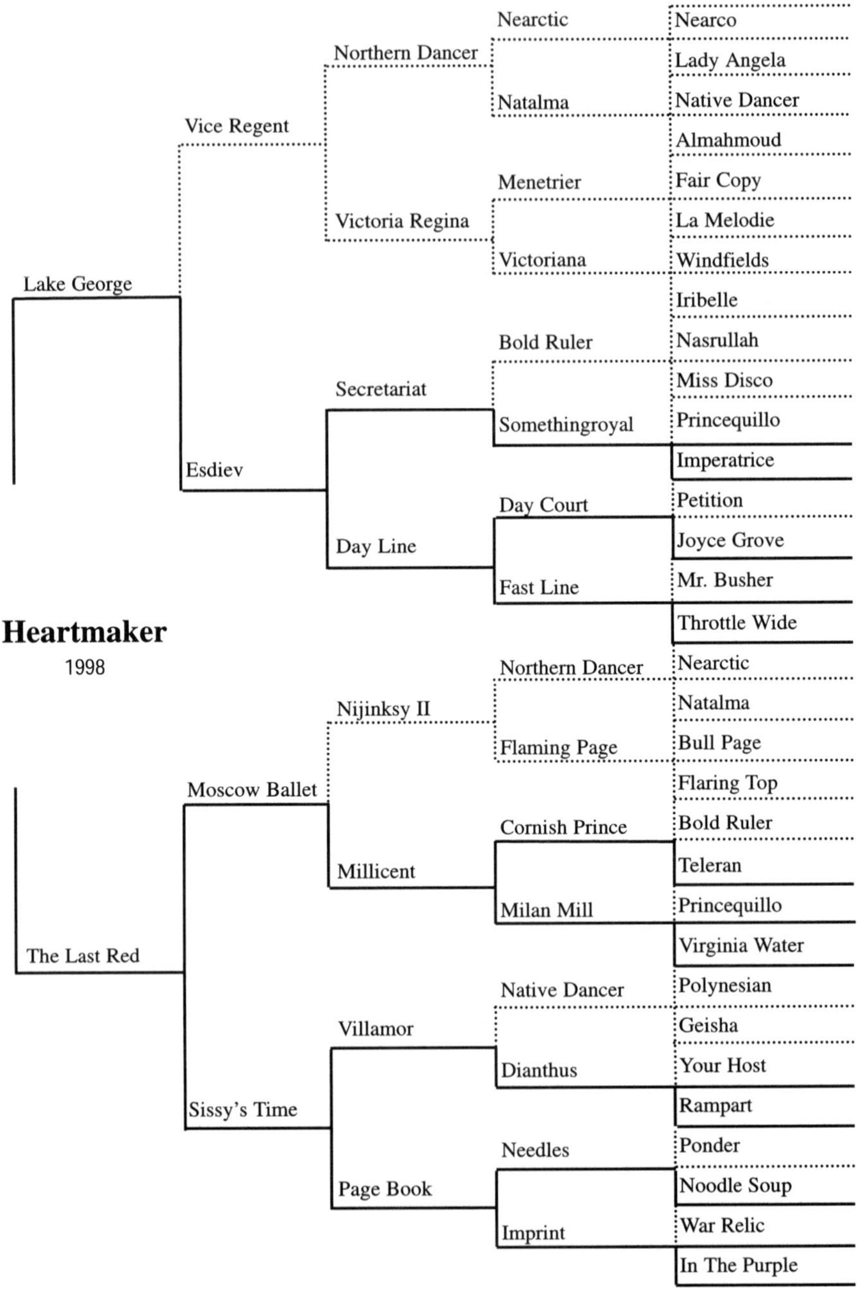

Tale of Two Hearts

1997

Parents	Grandparents	Great-grandparents	3rd generation	4th generation
Desert Secret	Sadler's Wells	Northern Dancer	Nearctic	Nearco
				Lady Angela
			Natalma	Native Dancer
				Almahmoud
		Fairy Bridge	Bold Reason	Hail to Reason
				Lalun
			Special	Forli
				Thong
	Clandestina	Secretariat	Bold Ruler	Nasrullah
				Miss Disco
			Somethingroyal	Princequillo
				Imperatrice
		My Charmer	Poker	Round Table
				Glamour
			Fair Charmer	Jet Action
				Myrtle Charm
The Last Red	Moscow Ballet	Nijinsky II	Northern Dancer	Nearctic
				Natalma
			Flaming Page	Bull Page
				Flaring Top
		Millicent	Cornish Prince	Bold Ruler
				Teleran
			Milan Mill	Princequillo
				Virginia Water
	Sissy's Time	Villamor	Native Dancer	Polynesian
				Geisha
			Dianthus	Your Host
				Rampart
		Page Book	Needles	Ponder
				Noodle Soup
			Imprint	War Relic
				In The Purple

Eclipse

1764

Parents	Grandparents	Great-grandparents	4th generation	5th generation
Marske	Squirt	Bartlett's Childers	Darley Arabian	Unknown
				Unknown
			Betty Leedes	Old Careless
				Cream Cheeks
		Snake Mare	Snake	Lister Turk
				Hautboy Mare
			Grey Wilkes	Hautboy
				Miss Darcy's Pet Mare
	The Ruby Mare	Blacklegs	Hutton's Bay Barb	Unknown
				Unknown
			Coneyskins Mare	Coneyskins
				Clubfoot
		Bay Bolton Mare	Bay Bolton	Hautboy
				Makeless Mare
			Fox Cub Mare	Fox Cub
				Coneyskins Mare
Spilletta	Regulus	Godolphin Arab	Unknown	Unknown
				Unknown
			Unknown	Unknown
				Unknown
		Grey Robinson	Bald Galloway	St. Victor's Barb
				Grey Whynot
			Snake Mare	Snake
				Grey Wilkes
	Mother Western	Son of Snake	Snake	Lister Turk
				Hautboy Mare
			Akaster Turk Mare	Akaster Turk
				Pulleine Arab Mare
		Montague Mare	Montagu	Unknown
				Unknown
			Hautboy Mare	Hautboy
				Brimmer Mare

Chapter 12

Following Eclipse's Path

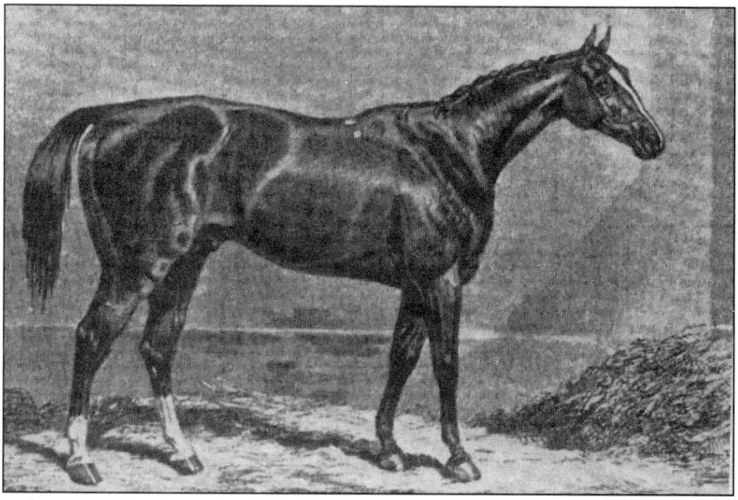

Painting by George Stubbs

Eclipse

Following the path of Eclipse's great heart has led to some interesting discoveries not only in terms of today's champions but where it came from in the beginning and how it has impacted the breed for nearly 300 years.

After realizing the genetic connection between Eclipse's great heart and the monster heart of Secretariat, many were curious as to where Eclipse got his heart. In trying to determine where it might have come from, the path seems to lead to his broodmare sire Regulus and then, following the X line, to his dam Grey Robinson, a daughter of Bald Galloway, out of a sister to Old Country Wench by Snake out of Grey Wilkes. Snake never raced because of a swelling on his leg supposedly caused by a snake bite in his youth, hence his name.

Research shows that Snake was out of a daughter of Hautboy. Hautboy was a son of Darcy's White Turk, imported from Aleppo in Syria in 1657.The problem with following the X through Hautboy is that the female side of his pedigree is lost in the mist of a history that paid more attention to the male line. It is possible to hypothesize that he must have had Middle Eastern blood on his dam side as well because his daughters, which would carry the X from his female side, follow the same pattern as other mares passing the large-heart mutation. Hautboy daughters are frequently found on the heartlines of the greatest of the early English sire lines.

The imported Middle Eastern blood came to England to give endurance to the horses being developed by the English aristocracy. Speed had been added to the English cobs from the Irish Hobby horses but breeders needed more endurance for longer races and for the battlefield. This came out of the East with infusions of Arab, Turk and Barb horses.

These breeds not only brought larger hearts but also greater airflow and more refined features to the Thoroughbred. Another characteristic which seems to come out of these breeds and follows the large heartline are small ears.

Without the ability to go back and measure the early horses, research has to look for similar patterns in early pedigrees and follow that pattern forward.The pattern of performance seen in today's Thoroughbreds carrying the large heart was apparent 300 years ago if only someone would have followed the female lines.

In looking at the pedigrees of the early foundation horses before Eclipse's time, it becomes apparent that there is a consistent pattern in the earliest horses. Horses like Herod, Matchem, Bartlet's Childers, Bald Galloway, Old Bald Peg, Squirt, Old Morraco Mare, Grey Hautboy, Bay Bolton and Regulus, to name a few, all carried Middle Eastern blood on at least one of their X lines. If the leading sires and dams aren't themselves Arabian, Barb or Turk, they have these breeds on their X lines.

Regulus, who I consider one of the most successful of these, passed his heart to many but most importantly to Eclipse, Highflyer and Messenger. Also known as Sweetlips, Regulus was bred by Lord Chadworth in England. The son of the Goldolphin Arabian was foaled in 1739. In his racing career he won 10 races, including nine King's Plates. He was leading sire in England eight times between 1754 and 1766.

The sires with great hearts sired great daughters which went on to produce outstanding sons and daughters. The stallions with the great hearts all made their way to the bottom of the pedigrees of future racing stars.

With no way to go farther back than Hautboy, it is interesting to look for the X pattern forward and to find that in early important foundation sires, if they didn't have Eclipse, they seemed to have Regulus, Snake, Hautboy, or an Arabian, Turk or Barb on the X line.

It is fascinating to study the early sires such as Highflyer and see the same pattern as seen in today's large-hearted sires, where they were praised more for their daughters than their sons.

The sex-bias, which still exists today, made breeders look for sons of great sires and not value the daughters as well. Because breeders focused on the Y chromosome, the mutation for the large heart did not flourish as much as it might.

If the early Thoroughbred breeders had followed the female lines as did the early breeders in the Middle East, then the large heart would be a common trait today and not one that is usually found in only about 28 percent of the population.

But the sex-bias towards sons affected all the breeds, including today's Arabs, the only modern breed carrying the mutation that has not been crossed with the Thoroughbred. The large heart mutation in today's Arabian breed has the same wide range from small hearts to very large hearts found in today's Thoroughbred horses. Because of that love of the son of today's mighty stallion, there is just as wide a range in heart size in the

Arabs as in the other breeds. In our measurements of Arabs, we have found hearts ranging from five pounds to 14 pounds.

Aiding the preference for colts was the ongoing struggle between short races and distance races. While large hearts can be found in sprinters, small hearts are rarely found in distance horses. And as the fad wavered between speed and distance races, so the demand for speed and distance sires changed.

In the 1600s, when the aristocratic breeders wanted to run longer distances, they started importing the horses from the Middle East to add staying power, which we now know meant adding the larger heart and greater air flow found in those breeds.

In the United States in the mid to late 1800s, distance horses were falling out of favor as shorter races were being run and speed sires were being sought. This affected two of Kentucky's most legendary sires, Lexington and Glencoe, who were considered distance sires. When breeders started to want horses for shorter races, these two sires were passed over by many breeders looking for pure speed. Because of this, these stallions were mated to other breeds such as the developing Quarter Horse, Standardbred, Saddlebred, Tennessee Walker and Morgan horses.

Thus the large-heart mutation was introduced into other American breeds. Lexington and Glencoe added heart, stamina and speed to these other breeds as well as to the Thoroughbred.

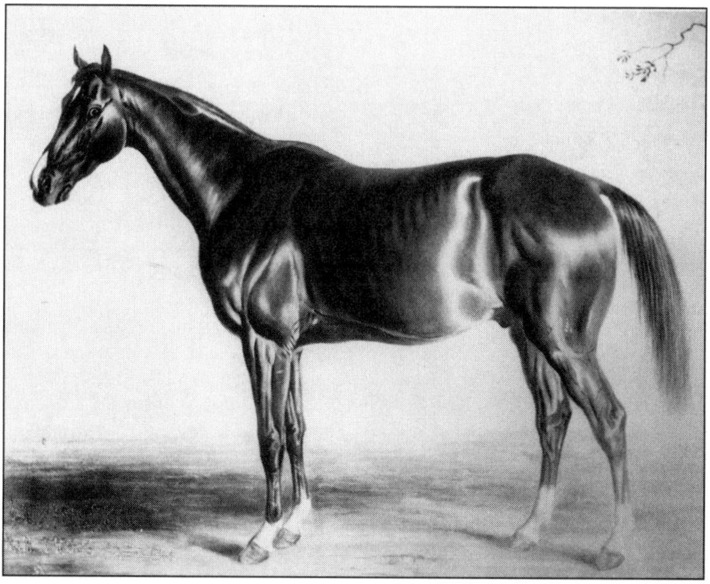

Painting by Edward Troye; courtesy of Grayson/Sutcliffe Collection

Lexington

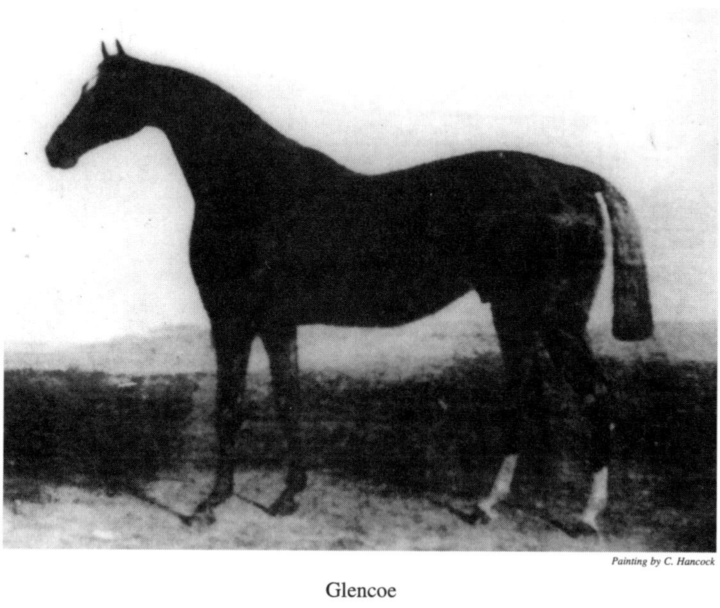

Painting by C. Hancock

Glencoe

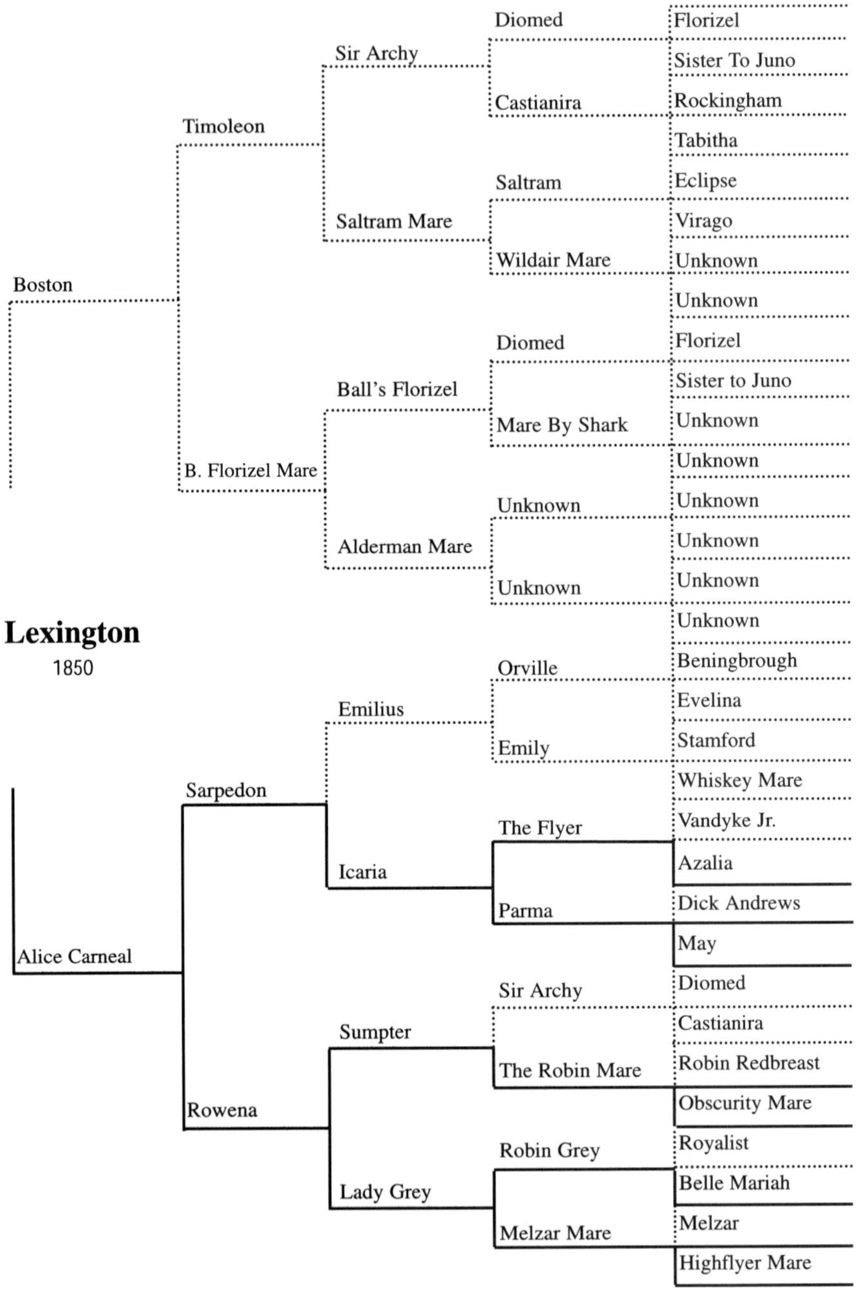
Lexington
1850
Boston
Timoleon
Sir Archy
Diomed
Florizel
Sister To Juno
Castianira
Rockingham
Tabitha
Saltram Mare
Saltram
Eclipse
Virago
Wildair Mare
Unknown
Unknown
B. Florizel Mare
Ball's Florizel
Diomed
Florizel
Sister to Juno
Mare By Shark
Unknown
Unknown
Alderman Mare
Unknown
Unknown
Unknown
Unknown
Unknown
Unknown
Alice Carneal
Sarpedon
Emilius
Orville
Beningbrough
Evelina
Emily
Stamford
Whiskey Mare
Icaria
The Flyer
Vandyke Jr.
Azalia
Parma
Dick Andrews
May
Rowena
Sumpter
Sir Archy
Diomed
Castianira
The Robin Mare
Robin Redbreast
Obscurity Mare
Lady Grey
Robin Grey
Royalist
Belle Mariah
Melzar Mare
Melzar
Highflyer Mare

Glencoe

1831

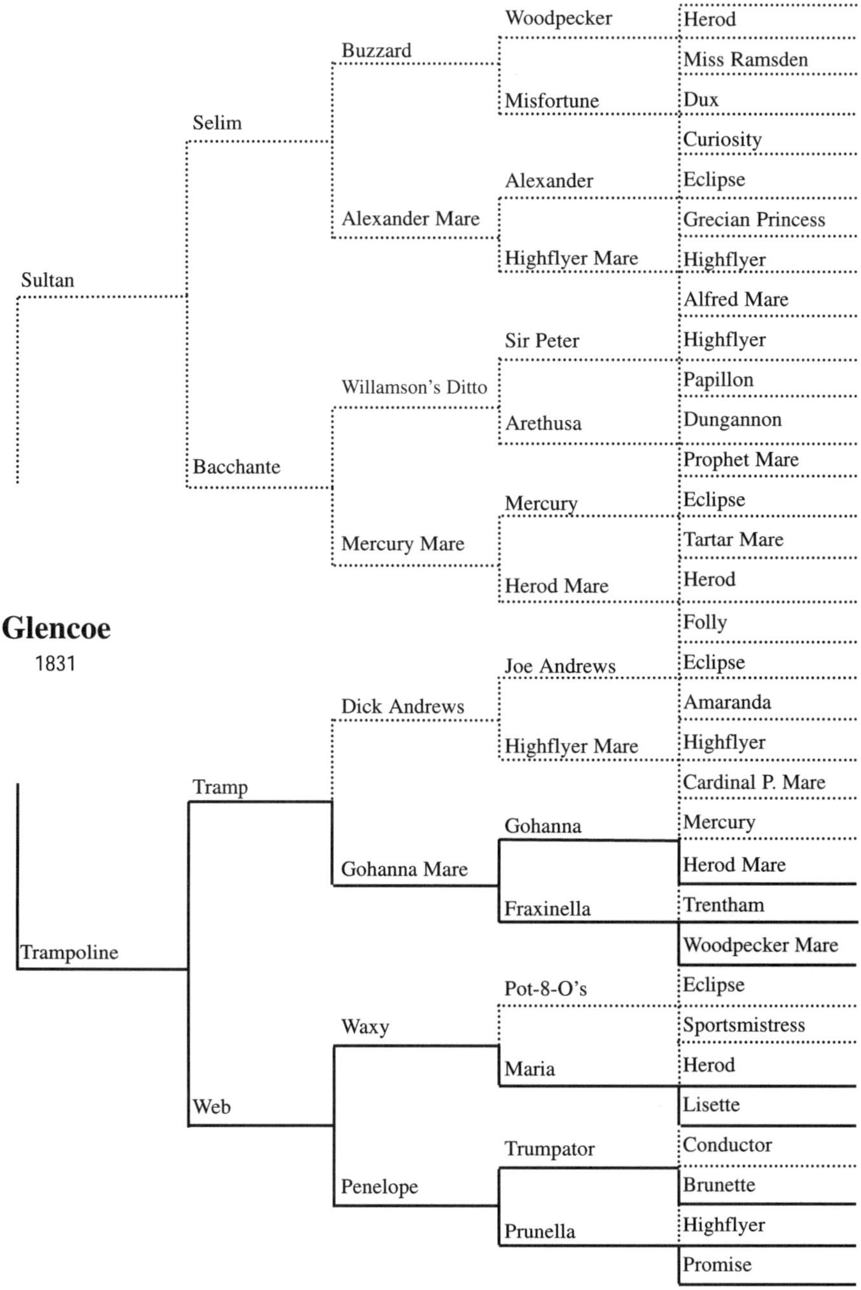

Highflyer Mare

1785

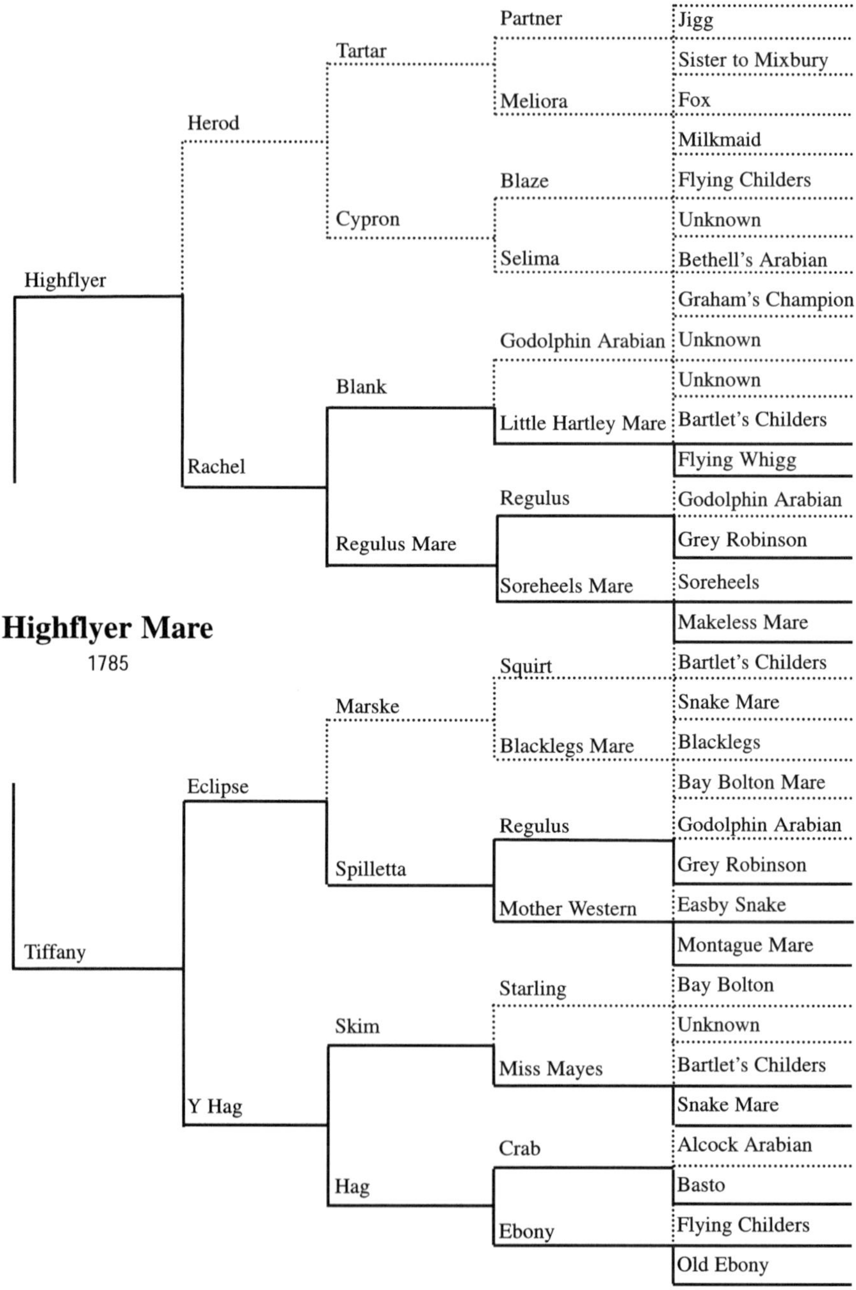

Chapter 13

Speed vs. Distance

Throughout the centuries the changing fad between speed races and distance races has had a dramatic impact on the development of the Thoroughbred breed. That and the sex bias in early and current breeders has led to some interesting situations and racehorses.

The old saw is that speed bred to speed will get you a short, fast horse. Distance bred to distance will get you a long, slow horse and speed bred to distance will get you a fast horse that can go a long distance. But it depends upon which X chromosome comes up. It is a matter of matching up the correct chromosome for the desired outcome. And Mother Nature can play some cruel jokes.

Speed obviously is desirable in a racehorse, but without a decent heart he may bloom early as a two-year-old and fall by the wayside at three when the races lengthen and the larger-hearted horses gallop by at the classic distances.

Breeding a speed sire to a distance mare has been the most successful combination. But even that can get tricky. A speed sire tends to have a normal-sized heart and likes distances from a sprint to a mile. Some can go up to 1 1/8 miles but not do the classic 1 1/4 miles or farther.

When bred to a mare with large heart lines, that sire's colts will be able to go the distance, especially if the mare is a double copy and always throws a large heart.

With the speed sire's daughters, it will be a matter of which X comes up. If she gets her dam's large heart and her sire's speed, she can be a world-beater. But if she gets her sire's heart and his speed, the best she will be is a sprinter. However, as a single copy she will be a good producer as long as she is bred to large-hearted sires.

One of the things a speed sire has going for him is that he will produce precocious two-year-olds so he will have early winners and attract better mares. The rule is the better the mares, the better the sons. And the industry judges a sire by his sons. To judge a sire successful, he needs sons that do even better than he did on the track. If he only ran six furlongs and didn't earn a tremendous amount, his sire record improves when bred to superior mares.

The heart grows until the horse is four and large-hearted individuals frequently take longer to develop. Cigar didn't make people sit up and take notice until he was four. In an industry graded by earnings, it is often the individual that has an early return of the money invested that gets the notice. But if you are on the Derby trail, that flashy two-year-old will fall by the wayside as the races get longer. That's when you need heart as well as speed.This is one of the reasons that many champion two-year-olds don't make it in the classics.

An example of a champion racehorse that combined great heart with great speed is Horse of the Year Holy Bull. He was considered the "people's horse" with his routine displays of brilliant speed and seemingly effortless races. Following his win in the Bluegrass Stakes, he didn't even seem to be breathing hard after running away from the field. When his owner-trainer Jimmy Croll would work him in the morning, his speed always surprised because it seemed so effortless. One did a double take when checking a stopwatch because it was hard to believe what it said when Holy Bull didn't appear to be putting out much effort at all. His only bad race in his three-year-old year was the Kentucky Derby, which has become the source of speculation about possible drug tampering by unknown individuals.

A true super horse, Holy Bull was measured and found to have a very large heart with a heart score of 147. The heart and body type he passes on his X chromosome is that of Blue Larkspur,

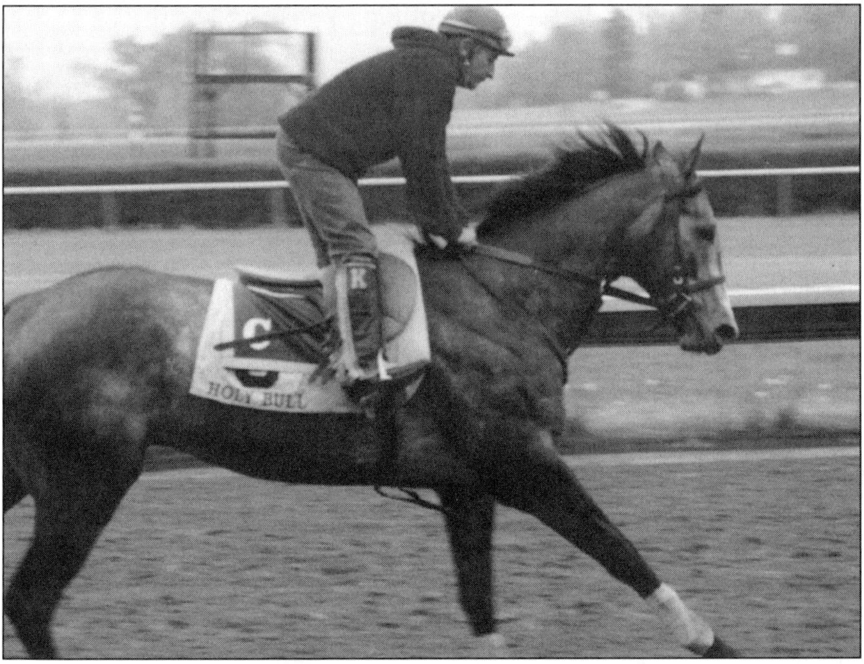

Photo courtesy of Marianna Haun

Holy Bull (Great Above X Sharon Brown)

one of the four super hearts, which he gets through his second dam Agathe's Dawn, a daughter of Grey Dawn. While Grey Dawn is out of a daughter of Mahmoud, he did not receive that X from his dam Polamia. Rather he got the Blue Larkspur X from Grey Dawn's third dam Blue Denim, a great broodmare by Blue Larkspur.

In a case like Holy Bull, when you find an extraordinary heart you look for its source in the pedigree. Without being able to measure horses already dead, you seek physical clues such as family resemblances to see which X may have come up. If you compare photos of Grey Dawn and Blue Larkspur, you see a striking physical resemblance in terms of body type and ears. The Mahmoud X is so distinctive in terms of the small round ears it passes that it is easy to see that neither Holy Bull nor Grey Dawn received that X chromosome. In addition, Holy Bull gets great speed elements from his sire's dam Ta Wee, half-sister to the brilliantly fast Dr. Fager. I don't believe that speed is a sex-linked characteristic and it can come from anywhere in the pedigree, top or bottom.

Holy Bull is already proving a success at stud, siring daughters like Confessional, who got his great heart, and sons like Macho Uno, Eclipse Award-winning two-year-old, who got his great speed. Holy Bull had a very big and very effective engine powering him around the track. And he was generally carrying an exercise rider who weighed around 150 pounds, a trick of trainer Jimmy Croll to help condition the colt for whatever weight he had to carry.

When you look at the offspring of a speed sire you will see better sons than daughters — just the opposite of the large-hearted sire who becomes known as a broodmare sire, with better daughters than sons.

Mr. Prospector was an outstanding example of a speed sire. He was by the speedy Raise A Native and had a normal-sized heart. He liked sprinting distances and only earned $112,171 dollars in 14 starts. This was an easy amount for his sons to trump.

But he had an amazing way of passing on speed to his offspring. He could give speed to his sons and his daughters, and he sired early winners that led him to the notice of the industry and brought him to Claiborne in Kentucky, the mecca of the Bluegrass. There he found superior mares and sired champion sons like Forty Niner, who inherited his sire's speed and his dam's heart.

Another champion son that benefited from the large-hearted mares with Claiborne connections was Woodman. Woodman inherited the large Buckpasser heart from his dam Playmate. He has been measured and has a heart score of 143, which is the War Admiral heart.

Seeking the Gold also carries the Buckpasser heart. These sires have been successful in not only passing on Mr. Prospector's speed but also their great hearts to their daughters.

Miswaki also carries the large Buckpasser heart line, but he expresses the Princequillo heart he inherited from his second dam Rose Bower, a daughter of Princequillo. He has the small curly Princequillo ears.

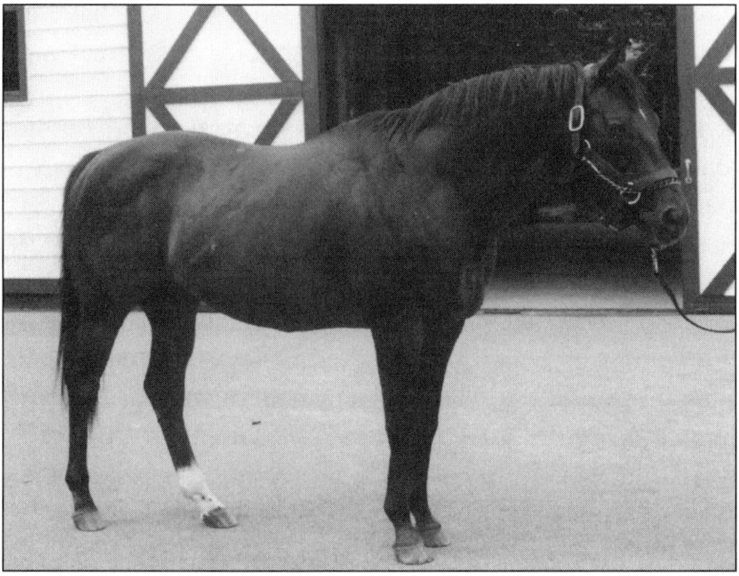

Miswaki

Photo courtesy of Marianna Haun

Galileo, the latest racing phenomenon from Europe and winner of the Irish Derby (Gr1) and English Derby (Gr1) in 2001, carries Miswaki's heart. Galileo was expected to face America's latest super horse, Point Given, in the $4-million Breeders' Cup Classic this year. Everybody was hoping that both horses would stay sound and be able to compete against each other. However, as often is the case in much-anticipated match-ups between great horses, injury interfered.

Following his dramatic win in the Travers Stakes (G1), Point Given was found to have a suspensory injury that would have taken quite a while to heal, and he was retired with earnings of just under $4 million. He had just won four (G1) $1-million races in a row and his potential hadn't yet been tapped, so it was quite a blow to racing and its fans. In winning his final race, Point Given had become the first horse since Damascus to win the Preakness, Belmont and Travers Stakes.

Point Given, who is by Thunder Gulch out of Turko's Turn by Turkoman, carries the heart and size of his broodmare sire. He stands more than 17 hands like Turkoman. They also have a similar head, ears and body type, although Point Given appears to have the speed, color and muscle of his sire. He should be a great sire, combining the speed of his sire and the heart of his dam.

Mr. Prospector, arguably one of the greatest speed sires of the 20th century, has sired extraordinary sons when mated to large-hearted mares. One of those sons, Fappiano, became a very successful sire himself, although he died relatively young. In Fappiano's pedigree, he allied Mr. Prospector's speed with the War Admiral heart of Dr. Fager. And when Fappiano was bred to Demure, a daughter of Dr. Fager, he sired Quiet American. Then, further inbreeding War Admiral, Quiet American was bred to another mare carrying the Buckpasser heart, courtesy of Believe It, and he sired Kentucky Derby winner and champion Real Quiet, who missed capturing the Triple Crown by inches. Fappiano also sired the successful sire Unbridled, who is out of a Le Fabuleux mare, and this seems to be the X he carries. Unbridled has sired Kentucky Derby (G1) winner Grindstone, champion Banshee Breeze, champion Anees, and Breeders' Cup Juvenile winner Unbridled Song, who is turning out to be a good sire himself. Aligning a successful speed male line with good heart lines on the bottom is working very well in this family.

Gone West is another outstanding son of Mr. Prospector who took the heart of Secretariat and allied it to the speed of Mr. Prospector. Gone West has sired such horses as English and French champion Zafonic, German champion Royal Abiar, Breeders' Cup Mile (G1) winner Da Hoss, millionaires Lassigny and West by West, as well as Belmont Stakes (G1) winner Commendable and Grand Slam, winner of $971,292.

Grand Slam was able to demonstrate his great heart when he was able to go on and be a graded stakes winner following a devastating injury he suffered in the Breeders' Cup Juvenile. He had already shown his talent at two by winning two Grade 1 races before the Breeders' Cup. Like his sire, Grand Slam combines the Princequillo heart he inherited from his maternal granddam Christmas Bonus with the speed of his Y line. He should be a great sire.

Another great son of Mr. Prospector, Conquistador Cielo, combined the great heart inherited from his dam K D Princess with the speed he got from his sire and won the Belmont Stakes, the test of champions.

All of these sons and many others have become successful sires passing speed to their sons and speed and heart to their daughters. They all illustrate what can happen when you breed speed to distance and the right X comes up.

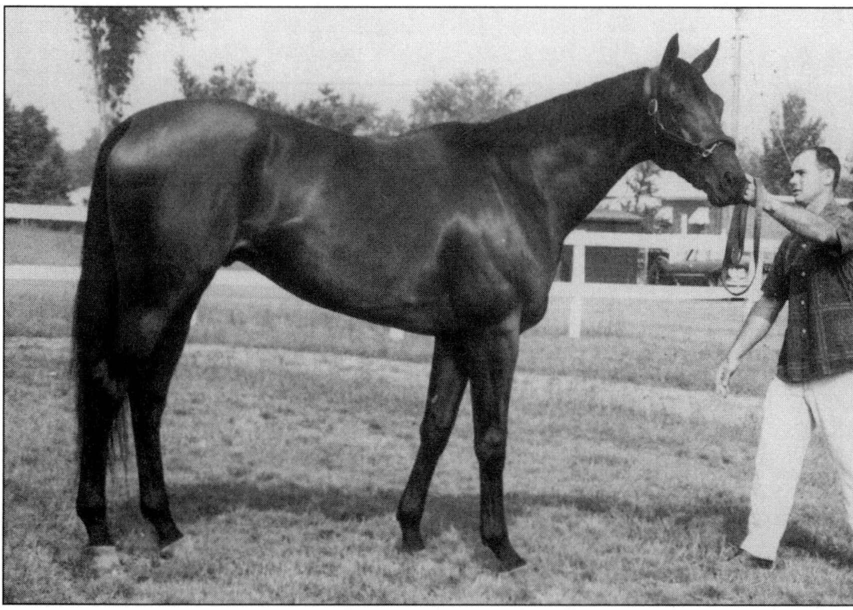

Photo courtesy of the Thoroughbred Times

Buckpasser (Tom Fool x Busanda)

Mr. Prospector
1970

- Raise A Native
  - Native Dancer
    - Polynesian
      - Unbreakable
        - Sickle
        - Blue Grass
      - Black Polly
        - Polymelian
        - Black Queen
    - Geisha
      - Discovery
        - Display
        - Ariadne
      - Miyako
        - John P. Grier
        - La Chica
  - Raise You
    - Case Ace
      - Teddy
        - Ajax
        - Rondeau
      - Sweetheart
        - Ultimus
        - Humanity
    - Lady Glory
      - American Flag
        - Man O'War
        - Lady Comfey
      - Beloved
        - Whisk Broom II
        - Bill and Coo
- Gold Digger
  - Nashua
    - Nasrullah
      - Nearco
        - Pharos
        - Nogara
      - Mumtaz Begum
        - Blenheim II
        - Mumtaz Mahal
    - Segula
      - Johnstown
        - Jamestown
        - La France
      - Sekhmet
        - Sardanapale
        - Prosopopee
  - Sequence
    - Count Fleet
      - Reigh Count
        - Sunreigh
        - Contessina
      - Quickly
        - Haste
        - Stephanie
    - Miss Dogwood
      - Bull Dog
        - Teddy
        - Plucky Liege
      - Myrtlewood
        - Blue Larkspur
        - Frizeur

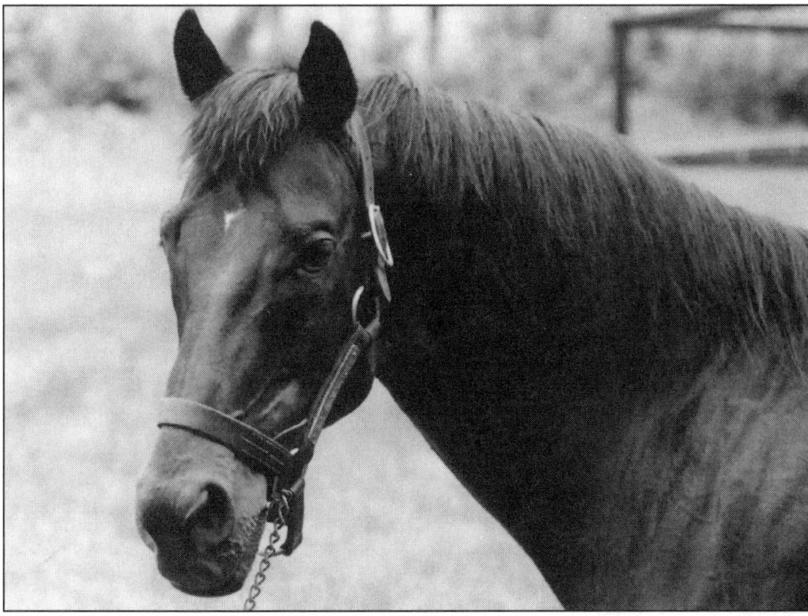

Photo courtesy of Marianna Haun

Mr. Prospector
(Raise A Native x Gold Digger)

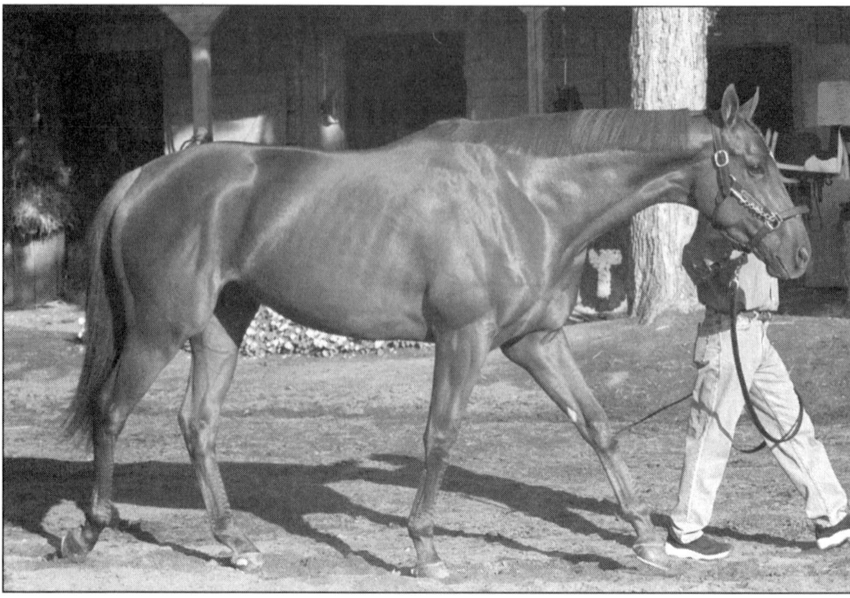

Photo courtesy of Patricia McQueen

Point Given (top) and Turkoman (bottom)

Photo courtesy of Patricia McQueen

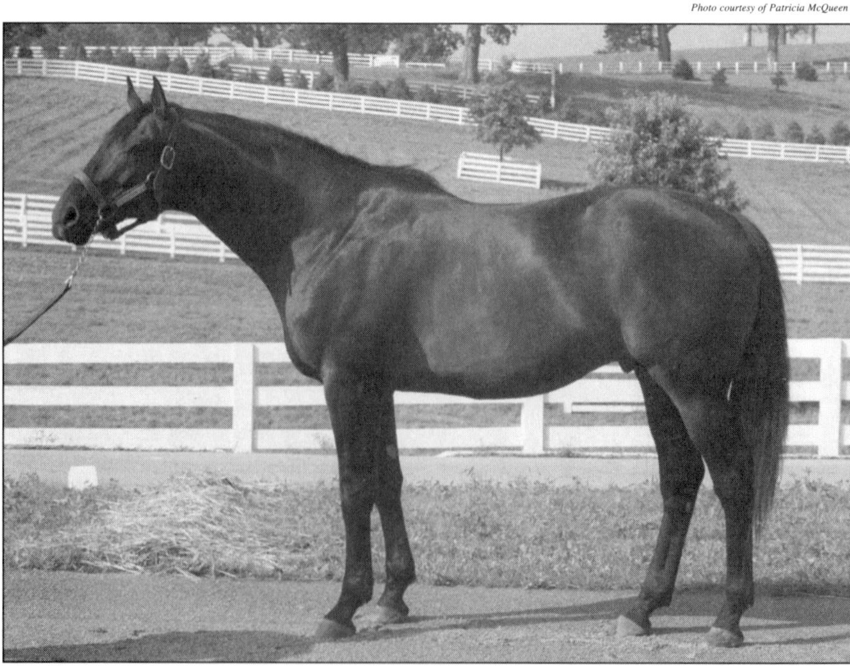

Point Given
1998

- Thunder Gulch
  - Gulch
    - Mr. Prospector
      - Raise A Native
        - Native Dancer
        - Raise You
      - Gold Digger
        - Nashua
        - Sequence
    - Jameela
      - Rambunctious
        - Rasper II
        - Danae II
      - Asbury Mary
        - Seven Corners
        - Snow Flyer
  - Line of Thunder
    - Storm Bird
      - Northern Dancer
        - Nearctic
        - Natalma
      - South Ocean
        - New Providence
        - Shining Sun
    - Shoot A Line
      - High Line
        - High Hat
        - Time Call
      - Death Ray
        - Tamerlane
        - Luminant
- Turko's Turn
  - Turkoman
    - Alydar
      - Raise A Native
        - Native Dancer
        - Raise You
      - Sweet Tooth
        - On-And-On
        - Plum Cake
    - Taba
      - Table Play
        - Round Table
        - Neallah
      - Filipina
        - Fomento
        - Rosa Roja
  - Turbo Launch
    - Relaunch
      - In Reality
        - Intentionally
        - My Dear Girl
      - Foggy Note
        - The Axe II
        - Silver Song
    - David's Tobin
      - Tobin Bronze
        - Arctic Explorer
        - Amarco
      - Restless Love
        - Restless Wind
        - Avignon

Turkoman

1982

- Alydar
  - Raise A Native
    - Native Dancer
      - Polynesian
        - Unbreakable
        - Black Polly
      - Geisha
        - Discovery
        - Miyako
    - Raise You
      - Case Ace
        - Teddy
        - Sweetheart
      - Lady Glory
        - American Flag
        - Beloved
  - Sweet Tooth
    - On-And-On
      - Nasrullah
        - Nearco
        - Mumtaz Begum
      - Two Lea
        - Bull Lea
        - Two Bob
    - Plum Cake
      - Ponder
        - Pensive
        - Miss Rushin
      - Real Delight
        - Bull Lea
        - Blue Delight
- Taba
  - Table Play
    - Round Table
      - Princequillo
        - Prince Rose
        - Cosquilla
      - Knight's Daughter
        - Sir Cosmo
        - Feola
    - Leallah
      - Nasrullah
        - Nearco
        - Mumtaz Begum
      - Lea Lark
        - Bull Lea
        - Colosseum
  - Filipina
    - Fomento
      - Guatan
        - Floretista
        - Guayaca
      - Fantine
        - Picapleitos
        - Fantasy
    - Rosa Roja
      - Rustom Pasha
        - Son-In-Law
        - Cos
      - Roseda
        - Fox Cub
        - Rosita Forbes

Fappiano
1977

- Mr. Prospector
  - Raise A Native
    - Native Dancer
      - Polynesian
        - Unbreakable
        - Black Polly
      - Geisha
        - Discover
        - Miyako
    - Raise You
      - Case Ace
        - Teddy
        - Sweetheart
      - Lady Glory
        - American Flag
        - Beloved
  - Gold Digger
    - Nashua
      - Nasrullah
        - Nearco
        - Mumtaz Begum
      - Segula
        - Johnstown
        - Sekhmet
    - Sequence
      - Count Fleet
        - Reigh Count
        - Quickly
      - Miss Dogwood
        - Bull Dog
        - Myrtlewood
- Killaloe
  - Dr. Fager
    - Rough'n Tumble
      - Free For All
        - Questionnaire
        - Panay
      - Roused
        - Bull Dog
        - Rude Awakening
    - Aspidistra
      - Better Self
        - Bimelech
        - Bee Mac
      - Tilly Rose
        - Bull Brier
        - Tilly Kate
  - Grand Splendor
    - Correlation
      - Free America
        - Blenheim II
        - Columbiana
      - Braydore
        - Roidore
        - Bray Beauty
    - Cequillo
      - Princequillo
        - Prince Rose
        - Cosquilla
      - Boldness
        - Mahmoud
        - Hostility

Gone West

1984

- Mr. Prospector
  - Raise A Native
    - Native Dancer
      - Polynesian
        - Unbreakable
        - Black Polly
      - Geisha
        - Discovery
        - Miyako
    - Raise You
      - Case Ace
        - Teddy
        - Sweetheart
      - Lady Glory
        - American Flag
        - Beloved
  - Gold Digger
    - Nashua
      - Nasrullah
        - Nearco
        - Mumtaz Begum
      - Segula
        - Johnstown
        - Sekhmet
    - Sequence
      - Count Fleet
        - Reigh Count
        - Quickly
      - Miss Dogwood
        - Bull Dog
        - Myrtlewood
- Secrettame
  - Secretariat
    - Bold Ruler
      - Nasrullah
        - Nearco
        - Mumtaz Begum
      - Miss Disco
        - Discovery
        - Outdone
    - Somethingroyal
      - Princequillo
        - Prince Rose
        - Cosquilla
      - Imperatrice
        - Caruso
        - Cinquepace
  - Tamerett
    - Tim Tam
      - Tom Fool
        - Menow
        - Gaga
      - Two Lea
        - Bull Lea
        - Two Bob
    - Mixed Marriage
      - Tudor Minstrel
        - Owen Tudor
        - Sansonnet
      - Persian Maid
        - Tehran
        - Aroma

Chapter 14

The Heart of Moscow Ballet

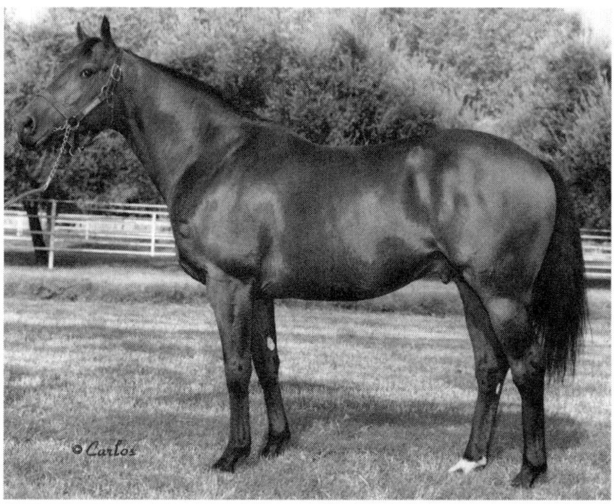

Moscow Ballet has literally been the heart of the X Factor project. In the course of the past six years, we have measured many sires and dams, yearlings, two-year olds and older racehorses all across the country. But it has been the horses of Harris Farms and the great heart of Moscow Ballet, his daughters and descendants that have provided us with our most in-depth knowledge about where the heart comes from, where it goes and how to breed for it.

We made our first visit to Harris Farms in California in the spring of 1996 where we measured Moscow Ballet and found the large Princequillo heart with a heart score of 147-150. That same morning, we measured the first Moscow Ballet daughter, Moscow Tap, who had his same heart score.

That mare now resides in Kentucky and is owned by William duPont III. Her 1999 son by Saint Ballado sold at the Ocala Two-Year-Olds in Training sale in February 2001 for $700,000. Her 1998 son Halo Strides by Strodes Creek has won close to $200,000 and was second to Balto Star in the 2001 $600,000 Spiral Stakes (G2) at Turfway Park in Kentucky.

Moscow Ballet, a graded stakes winner at two in Ireland, is a son of the storied Nijinsky II, out of Millicent by Cornish Prince. A half-sister to Mill Reef, Millicent's dam is Milan Mill by Princequillo. This is the heart that Moscow Ballet carries, and the same heart that was carried by champion Mill Reef.

Ironically, it is the same heart carried by Moscow Ballet's full-brother Western Symphony, who is making a name for himself as a broodmare sire in Australia.

Both sires are known for their daughters, the only ones capable of carrying their great hearts. In 2001, Moscow Ballet was in the national spotlight because of his multiple graded stakes winning daughter Golden Ballet, one of the leading three-year-old

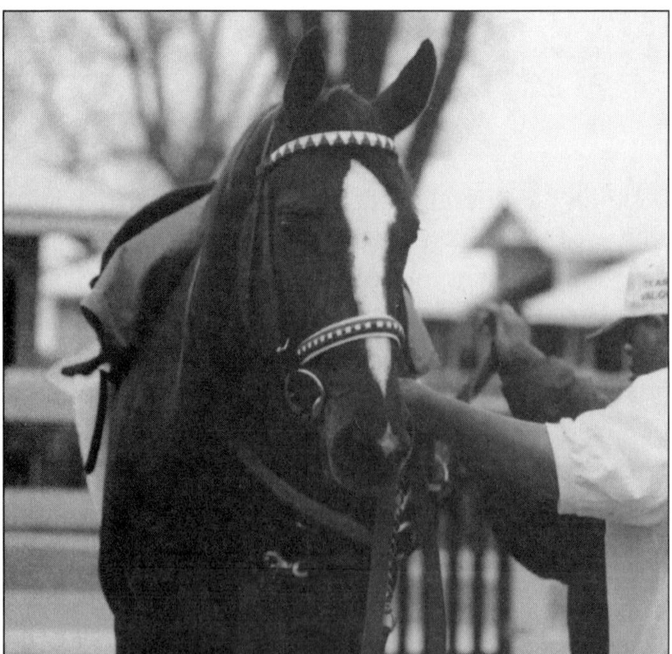

Golden Ballet, daughter of Moscow Ballet

Photo courtesy of Marianna Haun

fillies in the country.

In the spring of 2001, Golden Ballet won two Grade 1 events: the Santa Anita Oaks (G1) and the Las Virgenes (G1). She was second in the Ashland Stakes (G1) at Keeneland. She also won the Santa Inez (G2) and the Railbird (G2) before bowing a tendon

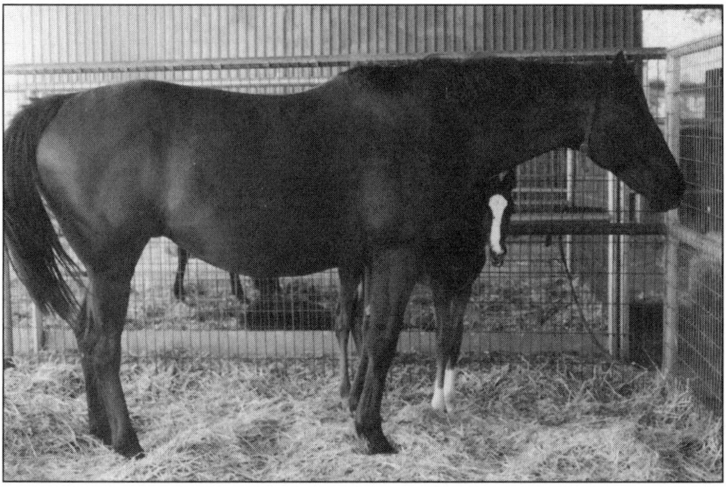

Photo courtesy of Marianna Haun

Soviet Problem, another Moscow Ballet daughter, and Escape With Me by Arazi

and retiring with earnings of $732,145 and a record of 10 starts with six wins, two seconds and two thirds. A blazingly fast filly, she was never out of the money.

She was very much like another Moscow Ballet daughter, Soviet Problem, who also got her share of national attention before she retired with earnings of $905,546 plus $60,000 from Japan. Soviet Problem participated in one of the most stirring Breeders' Cup Sprint races where she lost by a nostril to Cherokee Run at the wire after setting fractions faster than Secretariat's. Her gallant effort garnered her almost more praise from Turf writers than the eventual winner.

Soviet Problem was a wonder horse from California who couldn't find fillies fast enough to compete against and won two match races, one against a colt and one against a stakes-winning filly at Hollywood Park where she set a course record. She shipped across the country to beat the boys in the Laurel Dash (G3) on her way to the Breeders' Cup at Churchill Downs in 1994.

Although she won the California Oaks at a mile and a sixteenth, distance races were not her thing. She just couldn't wait. The gate would open and she was gone. She routinely ran six furlongs in 1:08.1 and 1:08.2. She would win her races by large margins, eight to 14 lengths, and the group in the winner's circle just grew and grew.

In 2001, she gave birth to a Quarter Horse son of leading sire First Down Dash (via a surrogate mare) and a Thoroughbred filly by Free House. While both foals are very good-looking, the son is a knockout and has the Princequillo ears so he should combine the speed of his dam and sire with the great heart of Moscow Ballet.

Moscow Ballet has progeny earnings of $13.8 million with an average earnings per starter of $34,966. He has also sired such daughters as Grade 1 winner Dominant Dancer, who earned $460,195 and won the Oak Leaf Stakes (G1) and the Landaluce Stakes (G3); graded stakes winner Teresa Mc, multiple stakes winner of $302,945; stakes winner Ballerina Gal, winner of $347,825; and stakes winner Leading Ballerina, winner of $230,139.

When bred to large-hearted mares he has sired sons like Moscow Changes, a stakes winner with earnings of $292,542, and Mr. Thrifty, a stakes winner of $243,743.

With 15 crops to his name, we have been able to follow his daughters and their offspring and confirm his large heart passing through four generations. We have followed it from him to his daughters and to their daughters and sons and to their daughters and sons.

We have taken a tiny twin daughter of his and bred her to four different large-hearted stallions and produced four different individuals, two daughters and two sons, with four different large hearts. The fillies expressed their sires' hearts and the sons each had a heart from one of her two X chromosomes. One daughter, Tale of

Two Hearts, carries the My Charmer heart and has a heart score of 147-150. Although it is the War Admiral heart, it is the same size as that of Moscow Ballet. Her second daughter, Heartmaker, who tragically died at two while in training, carried the large heart of her sire Lake George. Her first son Heart of Jaws by Huddle Up carries Moscow Ballet's heart. Her latest son, Man 'o Sheba by Alysheba, carries the heart of Man 'o War which came to The Last Red via her broodmare sire Villamor.

Villamor was out of Dianthus by Your Host, who has the Mahmoud heart and carries the small round ears that travel with that X. His second dam was Rampart, an amazing granddaughter of Man 'o War who made 104 starts, winning nine stakes races including the Gulfstream Park Handicap at 10 furlongs and the Black Helen at nine furlongs. She was out of the great Man 'o War daughter Boat. This was the X that Villamor passed.

This same X also found its way into the racing Quarter Horse world via the Thoroughbred Coup de Kas, who was out of a stakes winning daughter of Villamor, just as was The Last Red's dam Sissy's Time.

It was very nice of The Last Red to pass both her expressed and her recessive X to her two sons so that they could both be identified.

It has been a fascinating bit of racing trivia that the same Princequillo heart from his daughter Milan Mill has been fueling two outstanding fillies in two different hemispheres. While Golden Ballet dazzled in America, an even more extraordinary mare, Sunline, galloped on the world stage carrying the heart of her broodmare sire and Moscow Ballet's full brother, Western Symphony.

While we haven't measured the Australian champion Sunline, based on the physical characteristics she displays it is a pretty good genetic bet that the X chromosome she expresses comes from Western Symphony.

She not only looks like her maternal grandsire but also like Moscow Ballet and has the same curly Princequillo ears. When comparing conformation shots of Moscow Ballet and Western

Symphony, the family resemblance is startling.

Foaled in New Zealand at Pleasanton Stud near Cambridge, Sunline was a November 1995 foal by Desert Sun out of Songline by Western Symphony.

Because she was foaled in the Southern Hemisphere, her foaling date is the opposite of what it would be in America and the racing dates are in the fall, not spring.

But whatever the season, she got noticed from the moment she hit the track. She won all three of her two-year-old starts, winning her first stakes race in her third start.

When she came back at three she really started to burn up the track, winning five in a row. It wasn't until her ninth start that her streak was stopped when she finished second to Rosie O' War. But she evened the score in her next start when she defeated that filly.

Sunline truly became the people's favorite at Sydney in the AJC Doncaster Handicap, Sydney's 1,600 meter-championship event of the autumn. The crowd sent her off at odds of 10-9 and she ran away from the field in the $A1-million race to claim her second Group 1 win as a three-year-old. The Randwick totalisator at the track had to send out for more money to make the payout.

Because of her brilliant three-year-old season, Sunline was an early favorite for the $A1.8-million W. S. Cox Plate, Australia's weight-for-age championship race and the only Southern Hemisphere race in the Emirates World Series. She won in her usual front-running fashion, becoming just the fifth female Thoroughbred to win the Cox Plate.

At four, she ran again in the Cox Plate and came home again the winner by a record-tying seven lengths, joining the company of the legendary Phar Lap by winning back-to-back Cox Plates. Following the race, she received a standing ovation from the crowd.

An interesting bit of pedigree trivia in Sunline's bottom side is that she descends tail-female from Phar Lap's dam Entreaty (1920) whose sire Winkie had as his third dam Hilarity, a daughter of Pocahontas's son King Tom.

With Sunline's second win in the Cox Plate, she became the first horse from the Southern Hemisphere to top $A6 million in earnings when she took her mark to $A6,334,691, outstripping champion Octagonal's record of $A5,829,231.

British Timeform ratings ranked Sunline the world's best turf mare for 1999-2000.

In her final race of 2000, Sunline reinforced her claim to "world's greatest mare." Showing a world of class, she overcame an arduous flight to Hong Kong, the changes in climate and the effects of a long campaign to win the G1 $HK10-million Hong Kong Mile race against a top international field, leading all the way.

In 2001 Sunline became only the second horse in the 33-year history of the awards to be named Horse of the Year in Australia twice. The honor marked the seventh time in the last 10 years that a horse bred in New Zealand took home Australia's top honor. In addition to Horse of the Year, Sunline was voted champion filly/mare and champion middle distance horse. In 2001, she is on track to try and capture her third Cox Plate.

It will be fascinating to see what Sunline and Golden Ballet will produce with all the speed and heart they can send to their offspring.

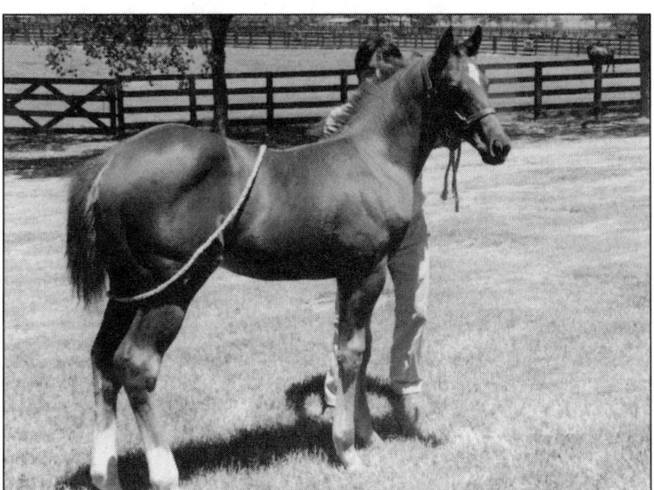

Soviet Problem colt, by First Down Dash

Photo courtesy of Bonnie Vessels

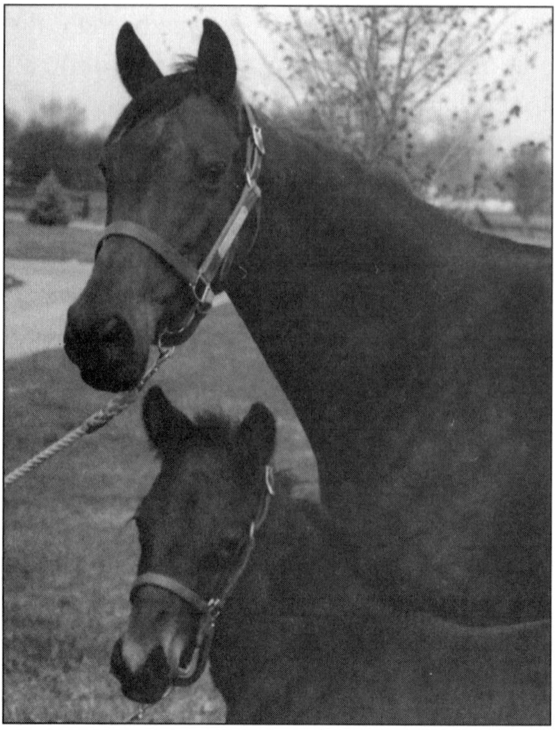

Moscow Tap and her 2001 colt

Photo courtesy of Marianna Haun

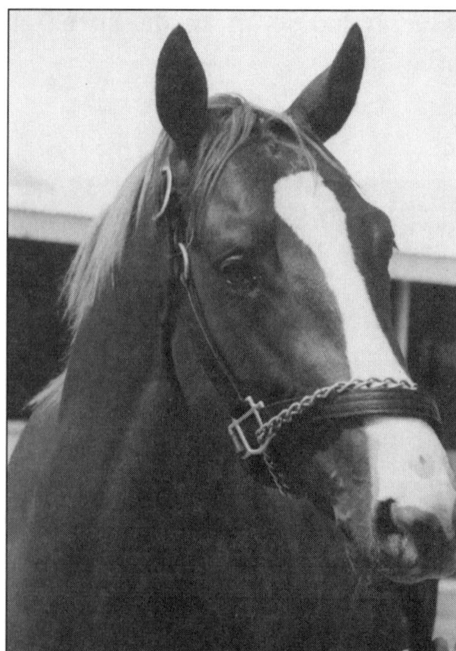

Axis, out of Moscow Tap

Photo courtesy of Marianna Haun

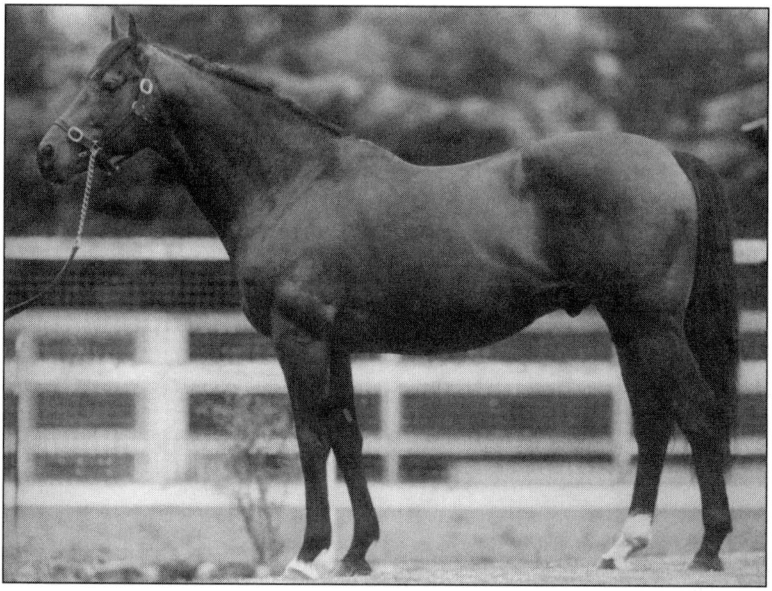

Photo courtesy of Mike Becker

Western Symphony

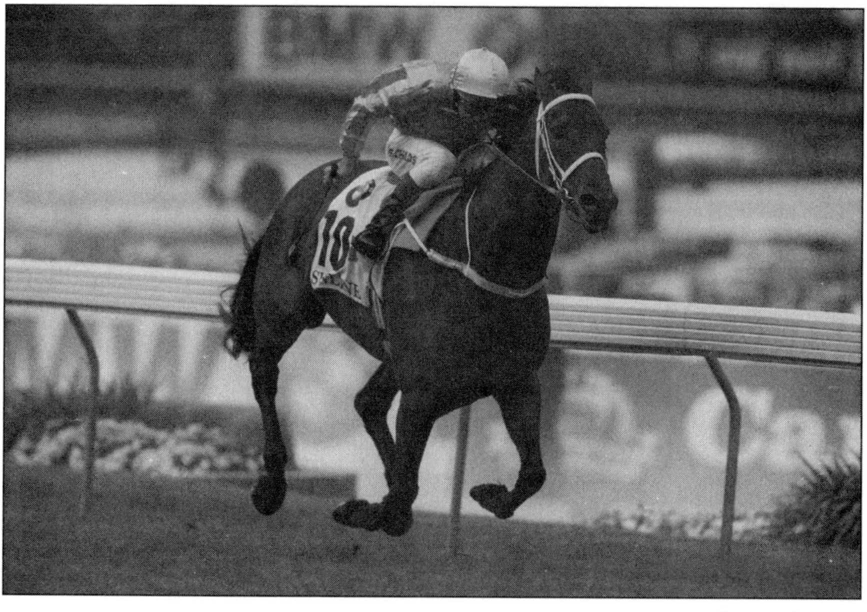

Photo courtesy of Martin King

Sunline

Messenger

1780

- Mambrino
  - Engineer
    - Sampson
      - Blaze
        - Flying Childers
        - Unknown
      - Hip Mare
        - Unknown
        - Unknown
    - Y Greyhound Mare
      - Y Greyhound
        - Unknown
        - Unknown
      - Mare By Curwen Bay Barb
        - Curwen Bay Barb
        - Unknown
  - Cade Mare
    - Cade
      - Godolphin Arabian
        - Unknown
        - Unknown
      - Roxanna
        - Unknown
        - Chanter's Sister
    - Little John Mare
      - Little John
        - Partner
        - Grey Brocklesby
      - Favourite
        - Unknown
        - Unknown
- Turf Mare
  - Turf
    - Matchem
      - Cade
        - Godolphin Arabian
        - Roxanna
      - Partner Mare
        - Partner
        - Bonny Lass
    - Daughter of Ancaster Starling
      - Ancaster Starling
        - Starling
        - Ringbone
      - Romp
        - Oxford Grey Turk
        - Ancaster Merlin Mare
  - Regulus Mare
    - Regulus
      - Godolphin Arabian
        - Unknown
        - Unknown
      - Grey Robinson
        - Bald Galloway
        - Snake Mare
    - Bolton Starling Mare
      - Bolton Starling
        - Bay Bolton
        - Mare By Son of Brownlow Turk
      - Snap's Dam
        - Fox
        - Gipsey

Chapter 15

In the Beginning There Was Messenger

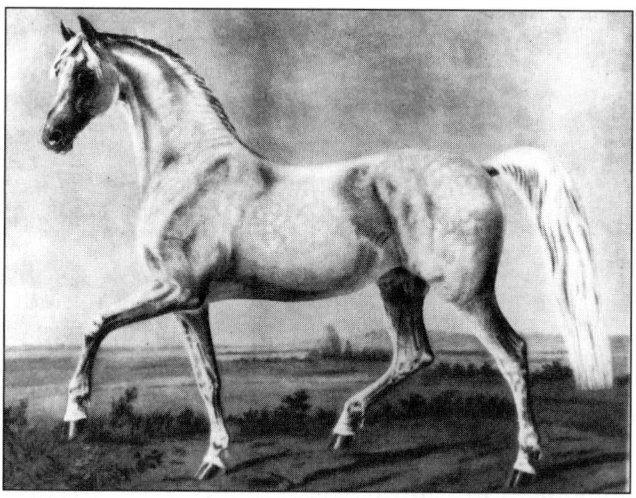

Photo courtesy of the Grayson/Sutcliffe Collection

Messenger

The Thoroughbred Messenger, who is considered the founder of the modern Standardbred, carried the same genetic mutation for the large heart from Regulus as Eclipse. He sent it down through his daughters where it ended up on a heartline in the legendary Hambletonian.

Messenger was foaled in England in 1780, the son of Mambrino out of a daughter of Turf, who was a son of Matchem. His second dam was a daughter of Regulus and he tracked on the tail-female line to a daughter of the Byerly Turk, his seventh dam.

The Middle Eastern influence is shown on most of the lines in his pedigree.

Racing from three to five, he won eight of 14 starts. Match races were the hottest tickets in England at the time and as he lost only one of the match races he participated in and gained forfeit in two others, he was probably a better racehorse than his record would indicate.

He arrived in Philadelphia from England in 1785 and stood his first year at stud there for $15 and spent the next 20 years with stud seasons in New York, Pennsylvania, and New Jersey. He died in 1808 at the age of 28.

It is ironic that it is not the sons of the mighty that pass on their greatness but their daughters. Every great heart finds its way down to the bottom of the pedigree where it is passed on from generation to generation. The pattern has been repeated and repeated for more than 300 years. The male line may die out but the heart continues.

The large-heart mutation was like a secret ingredient in the recipe for a great horse. It would be folded into the pedigree on the X line to appear and reappear in succeeding generations, producing horses some would describe as "freaks." It would always fall to the bottom of the pedigree to insure that certain individuals would inherit it and stand out in their generation. They would then find themselves in key positions in the pedigrees of future generations, occasionally appearing in a serendipitous manner to allow greatness to shine on a specific horse.

It started with Messenger, who brought the same large-heart mutation into the trotters that Eclipse brought into the Thoroughbreds through Regulus.

That large-hearted X found its way to the bottom side of the great Hambletonian and fueled his amazing career as a sire. Hambletonian's heart then went on to fuel the hearts of other succeeding trotters.

In Standardbreds, as with Thoroughbreds, the strongest pattern found in the best sires is to have speed on the Y (the tail-male line) and heart on the X. The stallion sends the Y to his sons and the X to his daughters. While not proven, there seems to be a pattern of speed from the Y and heart from the X on some of history's greatest racers, whether they are running on the flat or pulling a sulky. In Standardbred pedigrees tracing all the way back to Messenger, the large-heart mutation is found via Thoroughbred inbreeding. Once expressed in a sire or dam, that mutation is then repeated on the X lines of descending horses, particularly in the outstanding performers. Thus the pattern of performance seen following the X line in Thoroughbred racehorses is seen in successful trotters and pacers as well.

In Messenger's pedigree, you see his Y line going tail-male back to Flying Childers by the Darley Arabian. In Eclipse's pedigree, his Y line goes back tail-male to another Darley Arabian son, Bartlet's Childers.

It is interesting to note that both great sires combine a tail-male line to the Darley Arabian with an X line through Regulus, thus allowing them to send speed to their sons and heart to their daughters.

Ironically, Messenger is the sire of the dam of American Eclipse. American Eclipse was foaled in 1814. He was by Duroc and out of Miller's Damsel (1802) by Messenger. His second dam was a daughter of Eclipse's son, Pot 8 O's, out of a daughter of Gimcrack out of Snapdragon, a daughter of Snap, who was out of a daughter of Regulus. Historical hindsight can often be illuminating. Messenger's dam was an unnamed daughter of Turf out of a daughter of Regulus. Messenger was reportedly her only foal, and she passed her large-heart mutation to him which he passed to his daughters.

In the tradition of great-hearted sires, he found his way to the bottom side of the pedigrees of some outstanding horses, including the legendary Hambletonian, whose third dam Silvertail is a daughter of Messenger. That line is the strongest heartline found in his pedigree and the only one capable of producing the heart that could fuel the racing feats accomplished by the legendary trotter.

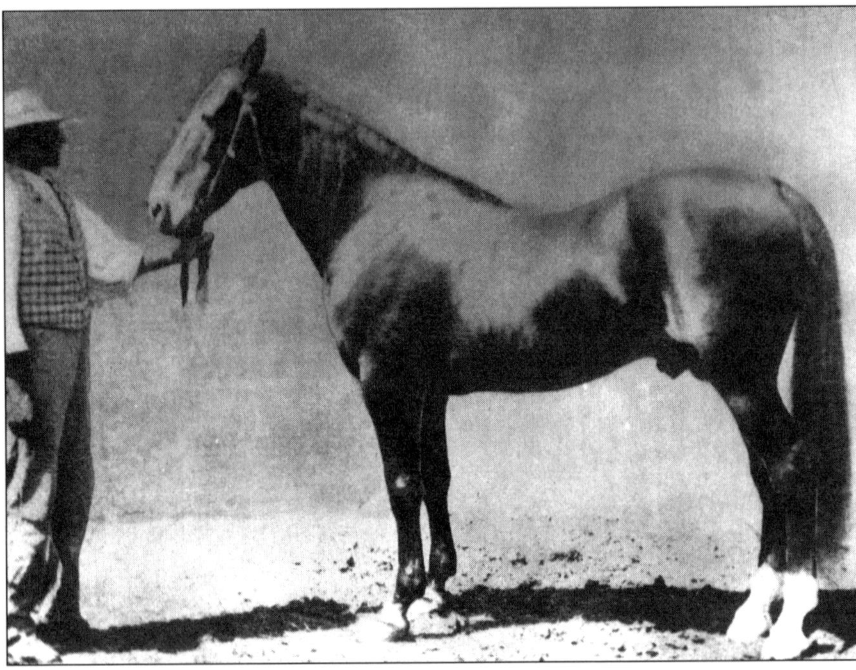

Photo courtesy of The Horseman and Fair World

Hambletonian

Chapter 16

Peter The Great

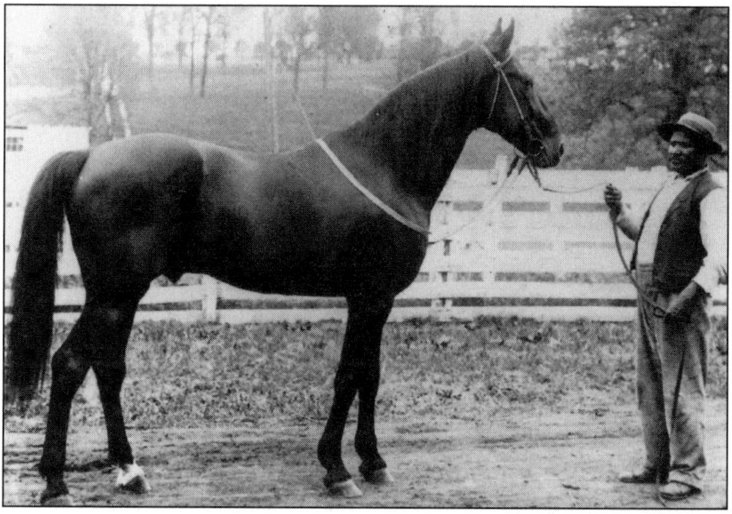

Photo courtesy of the Grayson/Sutcliffe Collection

Peter The Great

One of the greatest sires and broodmare sires in the history of Standardbreds is Peter The Great. He inherited the mutation from the Thoroughbred mare Brownlock, who traced back to Regulus on the X line through her sire Leviathan and through her dam, a daughter of Stockholder. Brownlock's second dam was a daughter of Pacolet, out of a daughter of Rosetta by Mendoza, whose second dam was a daughter of Regulus. Brownlock's fourth dam was a daughter of Ariel, who was out of a daughter of Regulus.

Following this pattern, Peter The Great passed his large heart into the pedigrees of succeeding generations of trotters, once again illustrating the idea that great hearts fall to the bottom of pedigrees and endure.

Foaled in 1895, Peter The Great was a great-grandson of the legendary Hambletonian. Through his sons Peter Volo and Peter Scott, his male family is found in nearly all of the major trotting lines today as well as a few pacing stars. A dominant broodmare sire, he is found on the X lines of such sires as Mr. McElwyn, Valley Victory, Spencer, Blaze Hanover, Star's Pride, Florican, Pine Chip, Mr. Lavec, Mack Lobell, Noble Victory, Speedy Crown, Speedy Scott, Super Bowl, the great gelding Greyhound and mares like Rosalind, Alma Lee and Helen Hanover, to name a few. His heart is on the X lines of great pacing sires as well, such as Albatross, Artsplace, Bret Hanover and Nihilator, among others.

Like all great broodmare sires, Peter The Great's heart is still making its way down the generations on the X lines in pedigrees today. Noted sire Mr. McElwyn is out of a daughter of Peter The Great. He in turn gave his heart to Star's Pride, who is out of a daughter of Mr. McElwyn. He is found on the X line of Speedy Crown via Florican and Mack Lobell via Speedy Count and Madge Hanover.

Artsplace, who earned more than $3 million, is the sire of $1.9-million earner Galleria, daughter of Emory Girl. Through his broodmare sire Albatross, he goes to such horses on the X line as Peter The Great, Volomite, Tar Heel and Spencer.

In her pedigree, Emory Girl traces to Midnight through Emily Ellen as well as to Volomite and Ethelwyn through On Time.

Without measuring the great sires, you can still get a good idea of their heart by their descent to the bottom of the pedigree of outstanding performers. That is the pattern of performance that so closely follows the large heart. It can be tracked on the racetrack and in the breeding shed. Great hearts will always be found on the X lines of history's greatest performers and producers. Another outstanding broodmare sire is Volomite, a grandson of Peter The Great, who goes to the Thoroughbred mare Esther by Express out of Coliseum by Colossus. Esther goes to Glencoe, sire of Pocahontas, on the X line through Colossus.

Peter The Great
1895

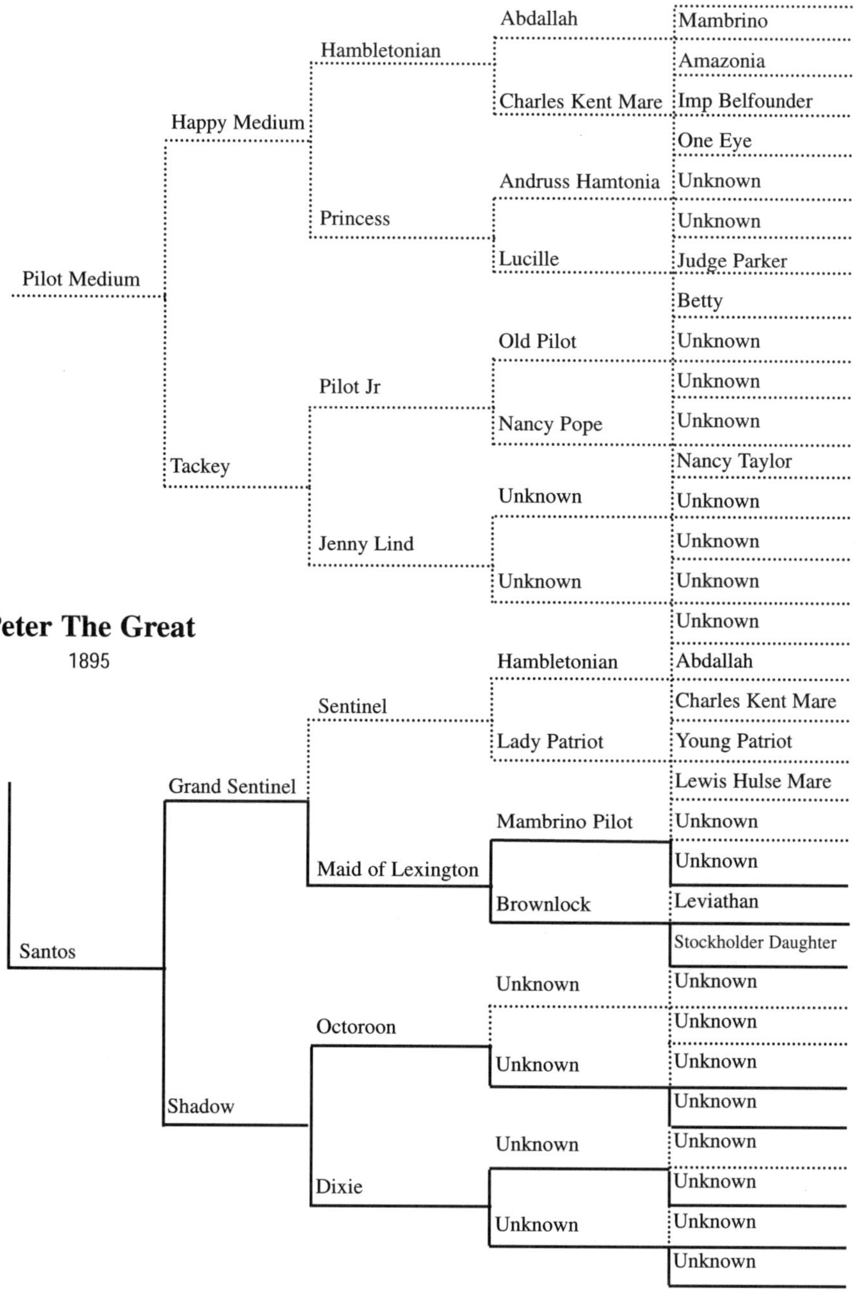

Volomite is found on the X lines of some of the greatest performers of the 20th century. He is a good example of what happens when a large-hearted sire is bred to a mare with a large heart on her X lines. Volomite was a leading sire and broodmare sire whose great heart also found its way to the bottom and influenced the hearts of other outstanding sires such as Tar Heel, out of Volomite's daughter Leta Long. We measured the heart of one of Tar Heel's daughters, Tarport Cheer, and found a large heart with a heart score of 133.

Tarport Cheer had zero earnings but has produced a number of outstanding foals, including Tarport Hap, by Most Happy Fella, who earned $688,664; Tyler B, also by Most Happy Fella, who earned $687,388; and Cheery Hello, by Albatross, who earned $869,619.

At Castleton Farm, we measured Flory Messenger, who was inbred to Peter The Great's grandson Mr. McElwyn through Blaze Hanover, Florican and Star's Pride. She had a very large heart with a heart score of 140. Foaled in 1978, Flory Messenger produced 13 foals. The best has been her first, a 1983 colt Express Ride by Super Bowl, who earned more than $1 million. Because he was a colt, it is certain that he was trotting with Flory Messenger's heart. She also produced the sire Carry the Message, by Royal Prestige, who earned $206,011.

With a horse like Peter The Great, it makes you think of that old Timex watch commercial — he has a heart that "just keeps on ticking" down generation after generation.

Flory Messenger
1978

- Arnie Almahurst
  - Speedy Scot
    - Speedster
      - Rodney
        - Spencer Scott
        - Earls Princess Martha
      - Mimi Hanover
        - Dean Hanover
        - Hanover Maid
    - Scotch Love
      - Victory Song
        - Volomite
        - Evensong
      - Selka Scot
        - Scotland
        - Selka Guy
  - Ambitious Blaze
    - Blaze Hanover
      - Hoot Mon
        - Scotland
        - Missey
      - Beverly Hanover
        - Mr McElwyn
        - Hanovers Bertha
    - Allie Song
      - Peter Song
        - Peter Volo
        - Evensong
      - Josephine Knight
        - Protector
        - Josephine Brewer
- Ball Belle
  - Florican
    - Spud Hanover
      - Guy Mckinney
        - Guy Axworthy
        - Queenly Mckinney
      - Evelyn The Great
        - Peter The Great
        - Miss De Forest
    - Florimel
      - Spencer
        - Lee Tide
        - Petrex
      - Carolyn
        - Mr McElwyn
        - Harvest Gale
  - Keystone Starlet
    - Stars Pride
      - Worthy Boy
        - Volomite
        - Warwell Worthy
      - Stardrift
        - Mr McElwyn
        - Dillcisco
    - Hostess
      - Bill Gallon
        - Sandy Flash
        - Calumet Aristocrat
      - Follow Me
        - Follow Up
        - Mimzy

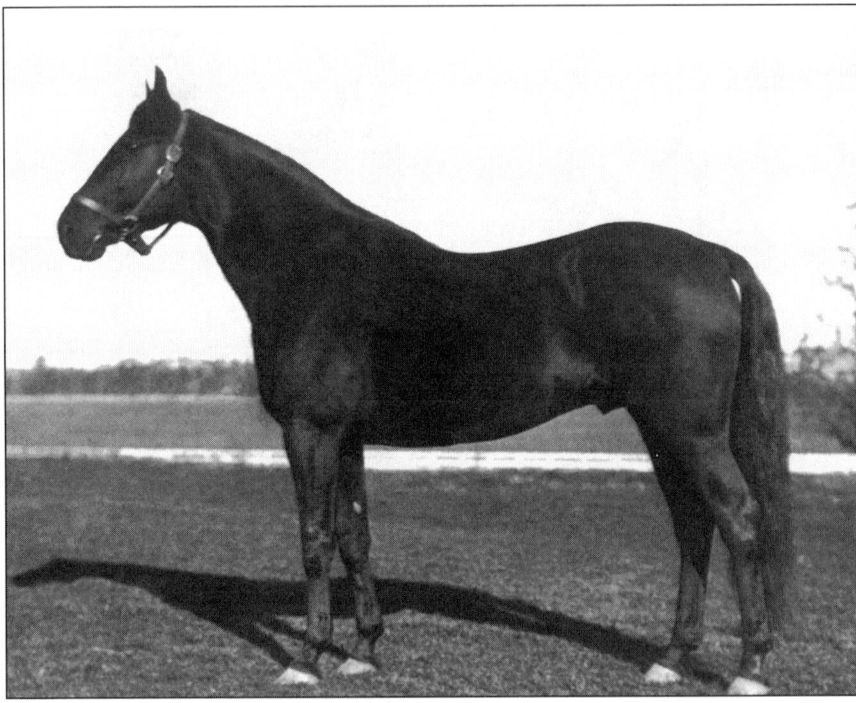

Photo courtesy of *The Horseman and Fair World*

Volomite, who is found on the X lines
of some of the greatest performers of the 20th century.

Volomite

1926

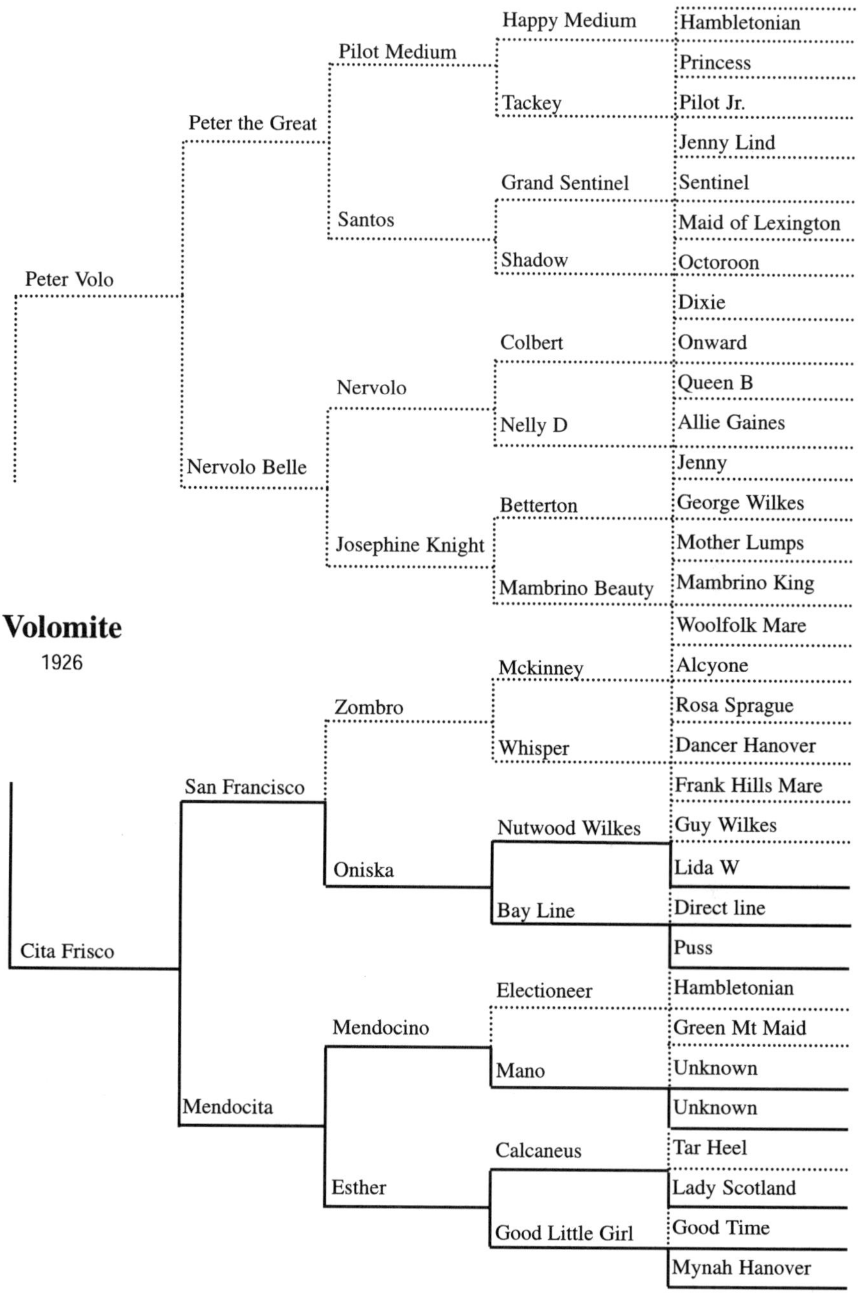

Galleria

1995

- Artsplace
  - Abercrombie
    - Silent Majority
      - Henry T. Adios
        - Adios
        - Greer Hanover
      - Hobby Horse Tar
        - Tar Heel
        - Wilellen
    - Bergdorf
      - Duane Hanover
        - Knight Dream
        - Dorsh Hanover
      - Princess Best
        - The Widower
        - Princess Chief
  - MissElvira
    - Albatross
      - Meadow Skipper
        - Dale Frost
        - Countess Vivian
      - Voodoo Hanover
        - Dancer Hanover
        - Vibrant Hanover
    - Ladalia Hanover
      - Columbia George
        - Good Time
        - Mitzi Eden
      - Lady Kacne
        - Duane Hanover
        - Lady Lunken
- Emory Girl
  - Sherman Almahurst
    - Royce
      - Albatross
        - Meadow Skipper
        - Voodoo Hanover
      - Sulta Rainbow
        - Tar Heel
        - Suave Hanover
    - Scuse Me
      - Majestic Hanover
        - Adios
        - Maggie Counsel
      - May C Byrd
        - Poplar Byrd
        - Poplar Topsy
  - Jodis Image
    - Striking Image
      - Strike Out
        - Bret Hanover
        - Golden Miss
      - Reflection
        - Painter
        - Way Wave
    - Little Jodi
      - Grand R
        - Unknown Sire
        - Unknown Dam
      - Maykirk
        - Darnley
        - Maytag

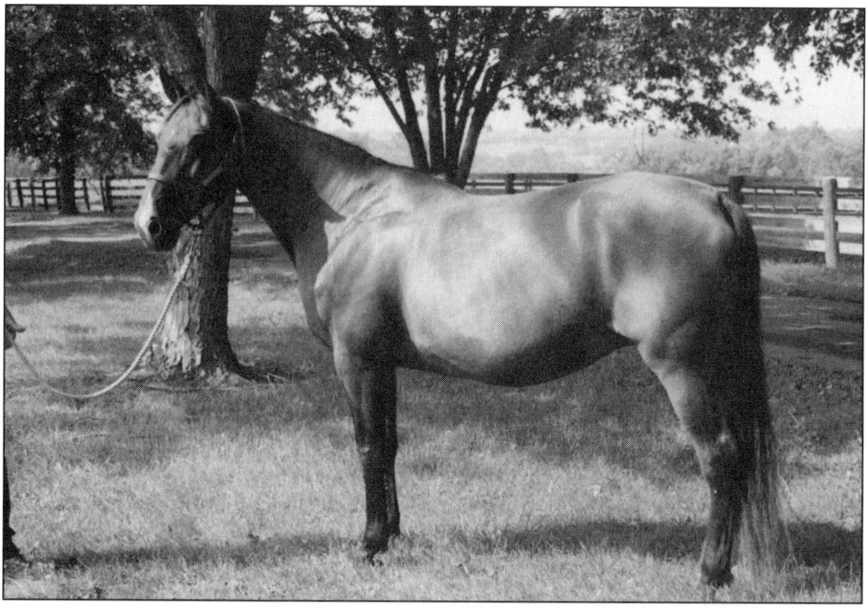

Photo courtesy of Marianna Haun

Emory Girl (top) and
daughter Galleria (bottom)

Photo courtesy of Kentucky Standardbred Sales

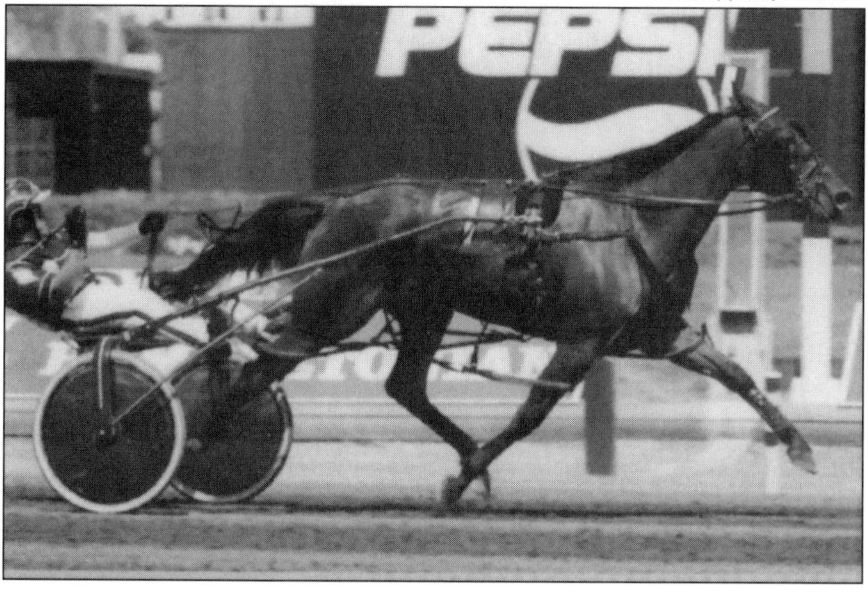

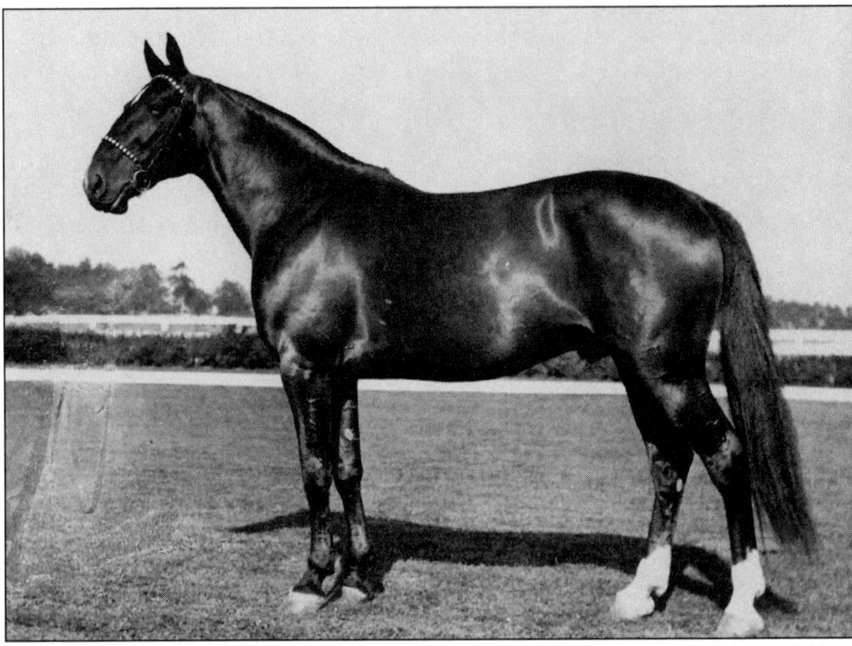
Photo courtesy of the Grayson/Sutcliffe Collection

Mr. McElwyn

Mr. McElwyn

1921

- Guy Axworthy
  - Axworthy
    - Axtell
      - William L
        - George Wilkes
        - Lady Bunker
      - Lou
        - Mambrino Boy
        - Bird Mitchell
    - Marguerite
      - Kentucky Prince
        - Unknown
        - Unknown
      - Young Daisy
        - Unknown
        - Unknown
  - Lillian Wilkes
    - Guy Wilkes
      - George Wilkes
        - Hambletonian
        - Dolly Spanker
      - Lady Bunker
        - Mambrino Patchen
        - Lady Dunn
    - Flora
      - Langford
        - Unknown
        - Unknown
      - Unknown
        - Unknown
        - Unknown
- Widow Maggie
  - Peter The Great
    - Pilot Medium
      - Happy Medium
        - Hambletonian
        - Princess
      - Tackey
        - Pilot Jr
        - Jenny Lind
    - Santos
      - Grand Sentinel
        - Sentinel
        - Maid of Lexington
      - Shadow
        - Octoroon
        - Dixie
  - Maggie Onward
    - Onward
      - George Wilkes
        - Hambletonian
        - Dolly Spanker
      - Dolly
        - Unknown
        - Unknown
    - The Widow
      - Wilton
        - Bye Bye Byrd
        - Beckilyn Hanover
      - Maggie H
        - Homer
        - Lady Sentinel

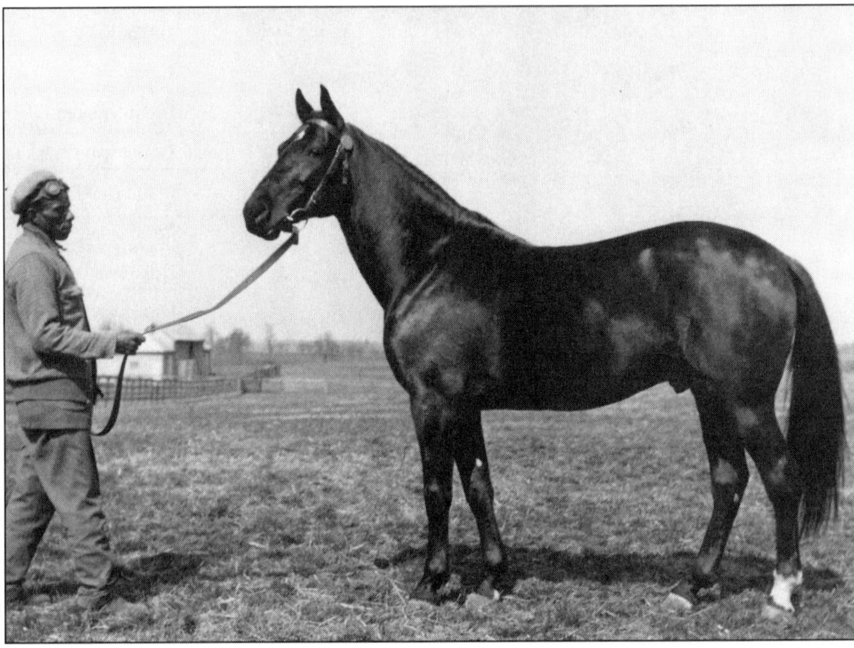

Photo courtesy of the Grayson/Sutcliffe Collection

Lee Tide

Lee Tide
1918

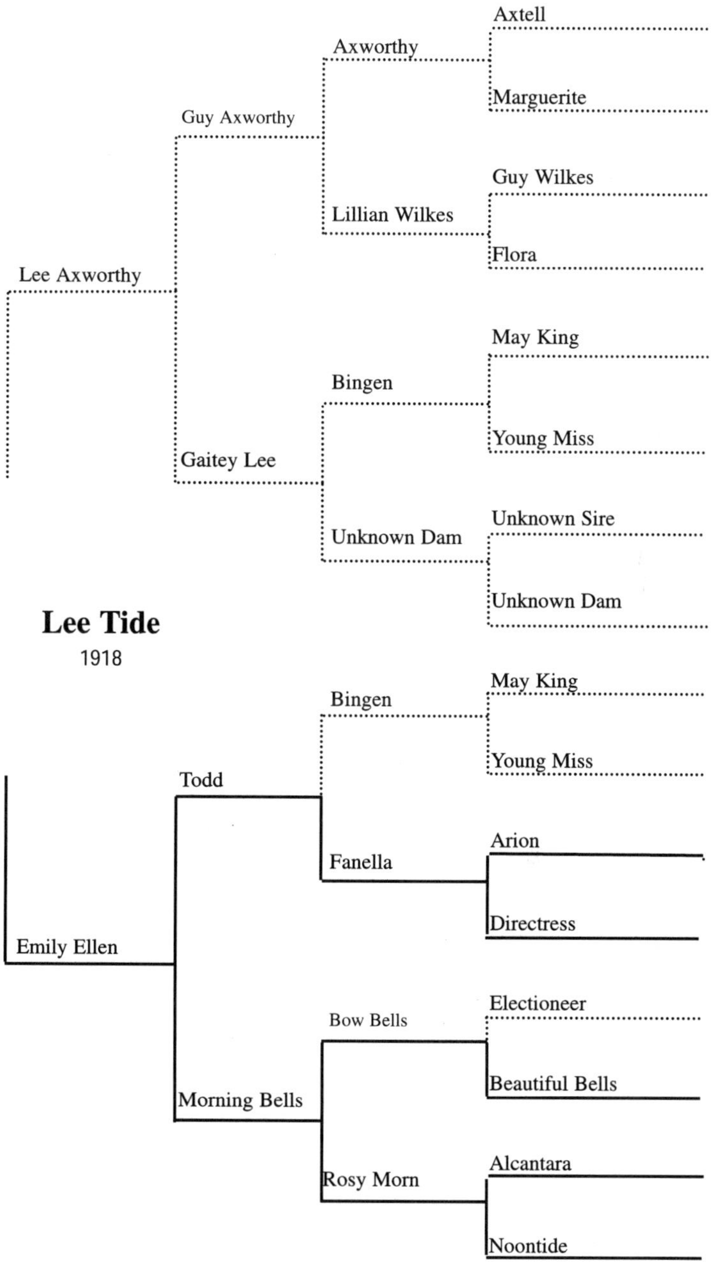

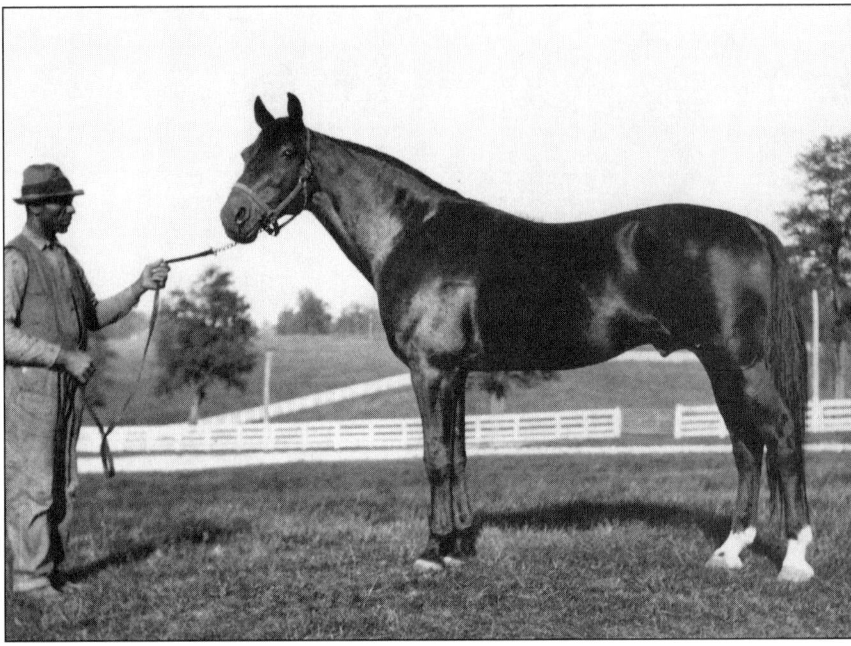

Photo courtesy of Grayson/Sutcliffe Collection

Belwin

Belwin

1910

Hambletonian

George Wilkes

Dolly Spanker

Alcyone

Unknown Sire

Alma Mater

Unknown Dam

Mckinney

Rhode Island

Gov Sprague

Belle Brandon

Rosa Sprague

Mabrino Messenger

Rose Kenny

Unknown Dam

Electioneer

Advertiser

Lula Wilkes

Adbell

The Moor

Beautiful Bells

Minnehaha

Belle Winnie

Hambletonian

Electioneer

Green Mt Maid

Gertrude Russell

Planet

Dame Winnie

Liz Mardis

Chapter 17

Maternal Influence

There have been several great female families that have passed the large-heart mutation down through generations of trotters.

Among the links in the large-heart line to Eclipse in the trotter's pedigree is a line that traces back to a mare named Midnight, foaled in Kentucky in 1865. She was out of a Thoroughbred mare that was a daughter of Lexington out of a daughter of Glencoe, sire of Pocahontas. Midnight and two other mares, Emily Ellen and Little Lie, who descend from her on the tail-female line, have had a profound influence on the best American trotters.

This maternal family is unique in that it is one of the few maternal families with two distinct modern branches. Emily Ellen's fourth dam is Midnight. Little Lie's fourth dam is Lady Kerner, who is out of Midnight and a half-sister to Noontide, Emily Ellen's third dam.

The two branches descend from half-sisters Noontide, foaled in 1874, and Lady Kerner, foaled in 1882. Both are out of the mare Midnight, who carries Eclipse's heart from her dam,Twilight, a daughter of Lexington out of Daylight, a daughter of Glencoe.

One of great broodmares passing Midnight's great heart is May Spencer, dam of World Champion and Hambletonian winner Spencer Scott and his full-sister Emily Scott, dam of Emily's Pride, a Hambletonian winner and Horse of the Year. Emily's Pride was the dam of Noble Victory, who is found in the same position on the X line of both Peace Corps and Continentalvictory.

May Spencer was a double-copy mare with large-heart lines on all of her X lines. She was intensely inbred since her dam and grandsire were three-quarter sister and brother. The actual crossing, as reported in John Bradley's *Modern Trotting Sire Lines*, is 3x2 to Emily Ellen and 2x4 to Guy Axworthy.

The Midnight line can be found on the X lines of the highest money earners in trotting history, including the all-time money earner Moni Maker, the richest mare in the world, who retired in 2000 with earnings of $5,589,256. She is also found on the X lines of Peace Corps, earner of more than $4.9 million, and sire Mack Lobell, earner of more than $3.9 million. Through her descendants, she has sent Eclipse's heart into the finest pedigrees in trotting history. Moni Maker is currently in foal to Valley Victory, who carries this same X line.

Great trotting sires also carry this X, mainly through the Emily Ellen line through her granddaughter May Spencer, her daughter Emily Scott, and her daughter Emily's Pride. Noble Victory is seen on the X line of outstanding modern sire Valley

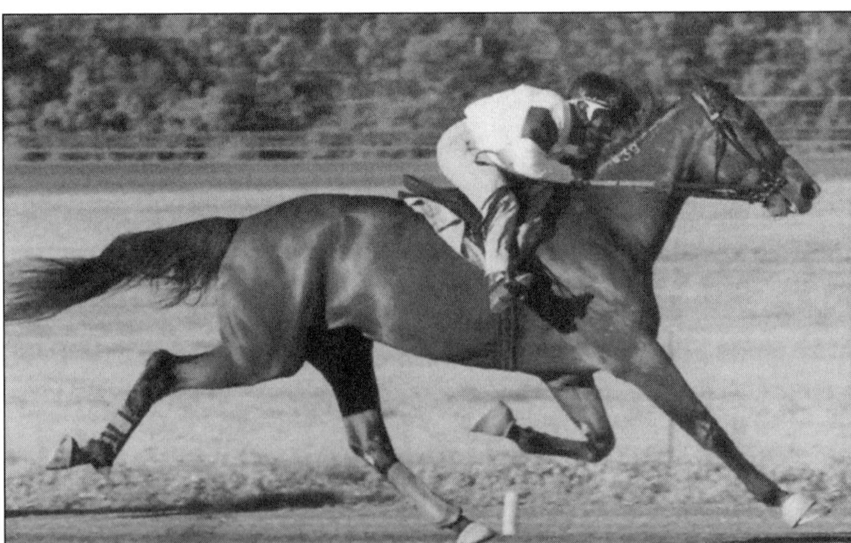

Photo courtesy of The Red Mile

Moni Maker, the richest mare in the world.

Moni Maker

1993

- Speedy Crown
  - Speedy Scot
    - Speedster
      - Rodney
        - Spencer Scott
        - Earls Princess Martha
      - Mimi Hanover
        - Dean Hanover
        - Hanover Maid
    - Scotch Love
      - Victory Song
        - Volomite
        - Evensong
      - Selka Scot
        - Scotland
        - Selka Guy
  - Missle Toe
    - Florican
      - Spud Hanover
        - Guy Mckinney
        - Evelyn the Great
      - Florimel
        - Spencer
        - Carolyn
    - Worth A Plenty
      - Darnley
        - Scotland
        - Fionne
      - Sparkle Plenty
        - Worthy Boy
        - The Gem
- Nans Catch
  - Bonefish
    - Nevele Pride
      - Stars Pride
        - Worthy Boy
        - Stardrift
      - Thankful
        - Hoot Mon
        - Magnolia Hanover
    - Exciting Speed
      - Speedster
        - Rodney
        - Mimi Hanover
      - Expression
        - Diplomat Hanover
        - Record Express
  - Nan Hanover
    - Speedy Count
      - Speedster
        - Rodney
        - Mimi Hanover
      - Countess Song
        - Victory Song
        - The Viscountess
    - Noble Nan
      - Noble Victory
        - Victory Song
        - Emilys Pride
      - Floriclaire
        - Floris
        - Claire Sampson

Victory, sire of Hambletonian winners World Champion Continentalvictory, 1996 Horse of the Year, and Victory Dream, three-year-old Trotter of the Year, to name a few of the many outstanding trotters, both male and female, he has sired.

Today Valley Victory is in a class by himself. According to John Bradley, he has taken over the leadership role of sires like Super Bowl and Speedy Crown.

It is interesting to note that both of those sires have links to large-hearted lines on the X chromosome. Speedy Crown goes to Peter The Great through Florican via Spencer and through Mr. McElwyn. Super Bowl's second dam Bewitch is a daughter of Volomite and his dam Pillow Talk goes tail-female to Peter The Great's daughter Evening Gale.

Valley Victory is following the path to greatness as a sire that Volomite, Star's Pride, Speedy Crown and Super Bowl traveled. All of these sires carried the Thoroughbred mutation in their pedigree.

It is impossible to know if all of these horses possessed and passed on the great heart that came into being through the Middle Eastern influence on the Thoroughbred more than 300 years ago. But it is possible to measure and find this great heart in the champion trotters and pacers today.

Other outstanding female families include Jessie Pepper, a mare foaled in 1861 with a strong Thoroughbred background that is verified in part and hypothesized in part. She carried a heartline to the Thoroughbred Sir Archy, who carried lines to the Darley Arabian and Snake, the source of Regulus's heart.

The Ethelwyn family is similar to the Midnight family. Ethelwyn's dam, Kathleen, the taproot mare, is by Pilot Jr. out of a Thoroughbred mare Little Miss by Sovereign, out of Little Mistress by Shamrock out of Glance. A look at the Thoroughbred lines in Little Miss are illuminating. Little Miss's sire Sovereign was out of Fleur De Lis who was by Bourbon, who was out of a daughter of Precipitate, out of a daughter of Highflyer, out of Tiffany by Eclipse. Fleur De Lis's dam Lady Rachel is by Stamford, who is out of Horatia by Eclipse.

Little Miss's dam Little Mistress is by Shamrock, who has lines to Highflyer and Everlasting by Eclipse. Her dam Glance is by Waxy Pope, who is out of Prunella, a daughter of Highflyer. Her dam Globe is by Quiz, who is out of Miss West by Matchem out of a daughter of Regulus. Globe's dam Paleface is by Young Woodpecker, who is out of a daughter of Eclipse, whose second dam is by Regulus.

So a strong pattern to the great heart of Eclipse is evident.

Another link between Midnight and Ethelwyn was the fact that Ethelwyn's sire Harold was an inbred son of Hambletonian, as was Noontide, the daughter of Midnight. Ethelwyn's great-granddaughter Nedda added in the Thoroughbred line to Esther, who goes to Glencoe, the sire of Pocahontas, through her dam Colisseum.

According to John Hervey in his book, *The American Trotter*, Nedda is a key mare in the family with the principal speed lines running through Pleasant Thought and her half-sisters, Petrex by Peter The Great and Ethel Volo by Binvolo. I think they also added the heart of Peter The Great through Petrex.

These examples illustrate a few of the great maternal families. They have been among the most successful and the pattern is clear in terms of the heart that was bred into the breed, thanks to mares like these.

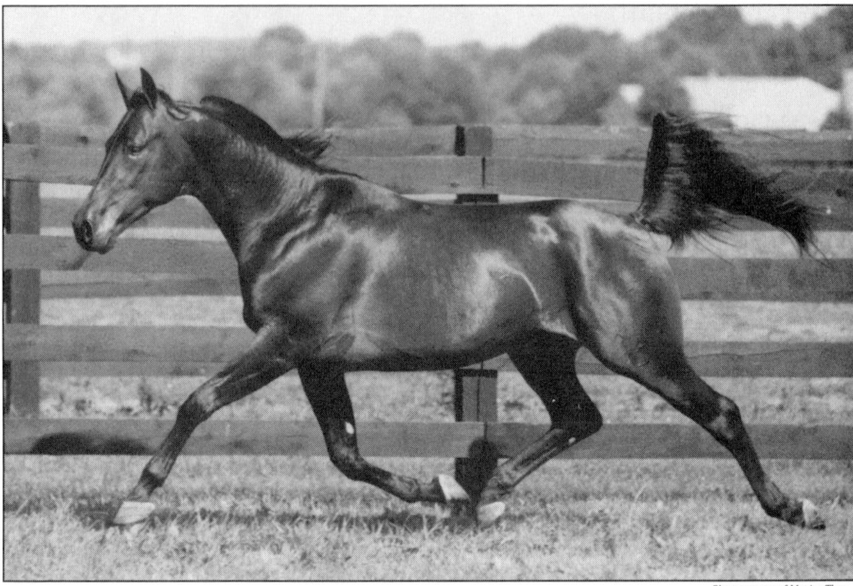

Photo courtesy of Monica Thors

Valley Victory

Valley Victory

1986

- Baltic Speed
  - Speedy Somolli
    - Speedy Crown
      - Speedy Scot
        - Speedster
        - Scotch Love
      - Missle Toe
        - Florican
        - Worth A Plenty
    - Somolli
      - Stars Pride
        - Worthy Boy
        - Stardrift
      - Laurita Hanover
        - Hoot Mon
        - Lark Hanover
  - Sugar Frosting
    - Carlisle
      - Hickory Pride
        - Stars Pride
        - Misty Hanover
      - Good Note
        - Phonograph
        - Rosemary Hanover
    - Karens Choice
      - The Intruder
        - Scotland
        - Mightly Margaret
      - My Tip
        - My Birthday
        - Lawful Tip
- Valley Victoria
  - Bonefish
    - Nevele Pride
      - Stars Pride
        - Worthy Boy
        - Stardrift
      - Thankful
        - Hoot Mon
        - Magnolia Hanover
    - Exciting Speed
      - Speedster
        - Rodney
        - Mimi Hanover
      - Expression
        - Diplomat Hanover
        - Record Express
  - Victorious Lou
    - Noble Victory
      - Victory Song
        - Volomite
        - Evensong
      - Emilys Pride
        - Stars Pride
        - Emily Scot
    - Lou Sidney
      - Darnley
        - Scotland
        - Fionne
      - Lucy Abbey
        - Guy Abbey
        - Princess Peg

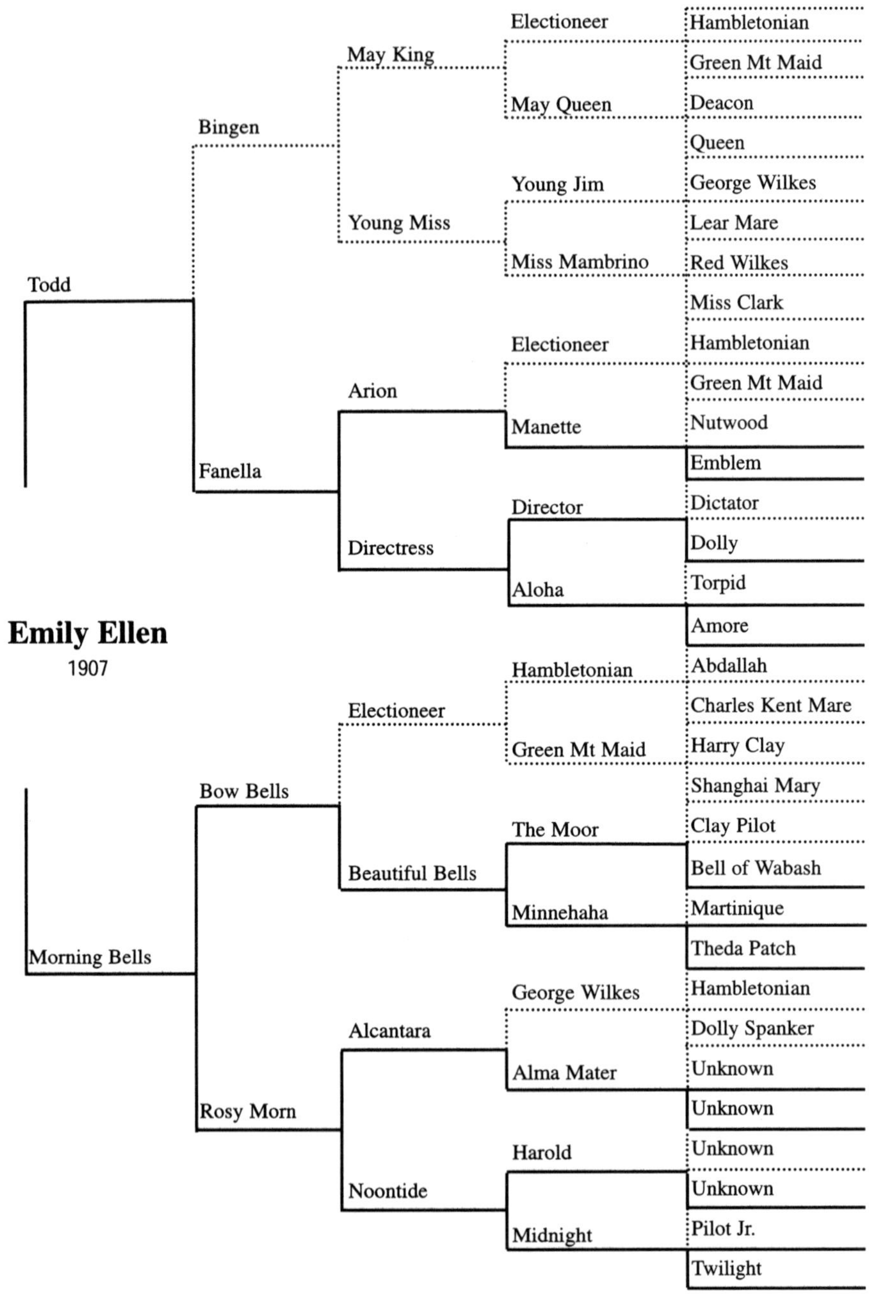
Emily Ellen
1907
Todd
Bingen
May King
Electioneer
Hambletonian
Green Mt Maid
May Queen
Deacon
Queen
Young Miss
Young Jim
George Wilkes
Lear Mare
Miss Mambrino
Red Wilkes
Miss Clark
Fanella
Arion
Electioneer
Hambletonian
Green Mt Maid
Manette
Nutwood
Emblem
Directress
Director
Dictator
Dolly
Aloha
Torpid
Amore
Morning Bells
Bow Bells
Electioneer
Hambletonian
Abdallah
Charles Kent Mare
Green Mt Maid
Harry Clay
Shanghai Mary
Beautiful Bells
The Moor
Clay Pilot
Bell of Wabash
Minnehaha
Martinique
Theda Patch
Rosy Morn
Alcantara
George Wilkes
Hambletonian
Dolly Spanker
Alma Mater
Unknown
Unknown
Noontide
Harold
Unknown
Unknown
Midnight
Pilot Jr.
Twilight

Continentalvictory

1993

- Valley Victory
  - Baltic Speed
    - Speedy Somolli
      - Speedy Crown
        - Speedy Scot
        - Missle Toe
      - Somolli
        - Stars Pride
        - Laurita Hanover
    - Sugar Frosting
      - Carlisle
        - Hickory Pride
        - Good Note
      - Karens Choice
        - The Intruder
        - My Tip
  - Valley Victoria
    - Bonefish
      - Nevele Pride
        - Stars Pride
        - Thankful
      - Exciting Speed
        - Speedster
        - Expression
    - Victorious Lou
      - Noble Victory
        - Victory Song
        - Emilys Pride
      - Lou Sidney
        - Darnley
        - Lucy Abbey
- Intercontinental
  - Chiola Hanover
    - Hickory Smoke
      - Titan Hanover
        - Calumet Chuck
        - Tisma Hanover
      - Misty Hanover
        - Dean Hanover
        - Twilight Hanover
    - Clorita Hanover
      - Stars Pride
        - Worthy Boy
        - Stardrift
      - Clorinda Hanover
        - Hoot Mon
        - Clotilde Anover
  - Pert Flirt
    - Noble Victory
      - Victory Song
        - Volomite
        - Evensong
      - Emilys Pride
        - Stars Pride
        - Emily Scot
    - Tosca
      - Speedster
        - Rodney
        - Mimi Hanover
      - Honor Bright
        - Bill Gallon
        - Rosalinda

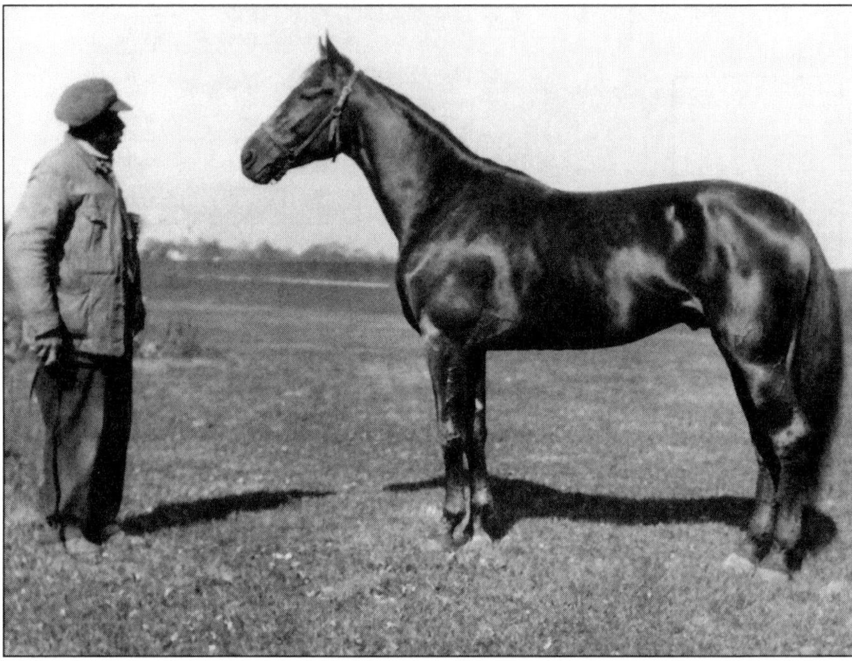

Photo courtesy of the Grayson/Sutcliffe Collection

Spencer, sire of May Spencer

May Spencer

1931

- Spencer
  - Lee Tide
    - Lee Axworthy
      - Guy Axworthy
        - Axworthy
        - Lillian Wilkes
      - Gaitey Lee
        - Bingen
        - Unknown
    - Emily Ellen
      - Todd
        - Bingen
        - Fanella
      - Morning Bells
        - Bow Bells
        - Rosy Morn
  - Petrex
    - Peter The Great
      - Pilot Medium
        - Happy Medium
        - Tackey
      - Santos
        - Grand Sentinel
        - Shadow
    - Extasy
      - Baron Wilkes
        - George Wilkes
        - Belle Patchen
      - Ethelwyn
        - Harold
        - Kathleen
- Guyellen
  - Guy Axworthy
    - Axworthy
      - Axtell
        - William L
        - Lou
      - Marguerite
        - Kentucky Prince
        - Young Daisy
    - Lillian Wilkes
      - Guy Wilkes
        - George Wilkes
        - Lady Bunker
      - Flora
        - Langford
        - Unknown
  - Emily Ellen
    - Todd
      - Bingen
        - May King
        - Young Miss
      - Fanella
        - Arion
        - Directress
    - Morning Bells
      - Bow Bells
        - Electioneer
        - Beautiful Bells
      - Rosy Morn
        - Alcantara
        - Noontide

Chapter 18

Trotters and Heart Scores

In first looking at racehorses with large heart scores, the Australians had seen a pattern of performance. This pattern indicated that horses with large hearts performed more successfully and consistently in the top races than horses with small hearts. Because of this observation, studies were conducted that involved both flat-racers and trotters, not only in Australia but abroad as well.

In the Denmark study of trotters by Nielsen and Vibe-Petersen of the Royal Veterinary and Agricultural University in Copenhagen, it was observed that there was a positive correlation between heart scores and earnings in races. The two Danish researchers recorded ECGs on 230 horses in training at Charlottenlund Trotting Track near Copenhagen.

According to their 1980 report, ECG recordings were made of seven horses over two years and on four horses over the following three years. Additional recordings were made in May 1970 of eight horses starting in the international race, the Copenhagen Cup. The recording method developed by Drs. Steel and Stewart was used.

After the ECG recordings were processed, Nielsen and Vibe-Petersen collected racing performance data from the Danish Trotting Society. All of the information, including the best kilometer time and the earnings, was fed into a computer for a statistical analysis.

Nielsen and Vibe-Petersen reported that heart scores increased with age and training. Yearlings were found to have an average heart score of 90 which increased to 110 by the age of five. They found a highly significant correlation between heart score and kilometer time in horses four years old and older, when the heart was fully grown. The level of significance was less in younger horses.

They found a positive correlation between earnings in races and heart scores. Horses with heart scores above 115 earned considerably more than horses with heart scores below this figure. The relationship was closer in stallions than in mares.

In terms of earning power, the 41 stallions with heart scores above 115 earned more than double what the 81 stallions with heart scores below 115 earned.

The relationship was not as well-defined in the group of mares studied. Mares with heart scores below 95 raced rather well compared with mares with higher heart scores. However, the small group of eight mares which had heart scores exceeding 115 had average stakes earnings that were considerably higher than the 45 mares with lower heart scores.

In the study of the eight elite international trotting horses competing in the 1979 Copenhagen Cup, the heart scores ranged from 124 to 152 which was considerably higher than the level recorded in the other horses that Nielsen and Vibe-Petersen found at a local trotting track in Copenhagen. Several of the horses competing in the Copenhagen Cup were ranked among the world's best trotters.

In the summary of their findings, Nielsen and Vibe-Petersen concluded that heart score is correlated with heart weight and is determined by a combination of heredity, age, growth and intensity of physical training. Their study confirmed and extended the data on heart score presented by Steel and his colleagues.

According to the report, "The results imply that a horse with a high heart score, i.e., a large ventricular myocardium, possesses a cardiac reserve of crucial importance for its qualities as a race horse.

"This may be due to greater myocardial strength and contractibility and to a greater distolic filling volume, resulting in a larger stroke volume. Bergsten (1974) measured minute volumes of 100 to 175 litres in horses trotting at submaximal speed on a tread mill. The cardiac output of a trotter racing at full speed is not known but it seems rather likely that a horse with a larger myocardial mass has an advantage over horses with a smaller cardiac reserve."

The researchers concluded that heart score appears to be a useful and simple indicator of racing potential in a trotting horse. They suggested it could be used as a screening device in young horses starting in training.

Heart Scores in Mares and Stallions of Different Age

Age	#	Mare Heart Score	SD*	#	Stallion Heart Score	SD*	#	Total Heart Score	SD*
1	4	90	nd**	4	93	nd**	8	91.3	13.8
2	19	92.9	12.1	33	99.5	9.2	52	97.1	10.7
3	26	98.4	11.7	37	107.8	12.6	63	103.9	13.0
4	17	97.7	12.4	34	108.4	11.9	51	104.8	13.0
>5	21	107.2	13.7	50	111.7	12.2	71	110.4	12.8

**SD = Standard Deviation* ***nd = not done*
(reprinted from the Equine Veterinary Journal 12 (2) 81-84)

Heart Scores and Racing Performance in Stallions and Mares

Heart score	Number horses	Average starts per horse	Average stakes per horse(DKr)*	Average stakes per start(DKr)
		Stallions		
<95	18	11	8,115	706
96-105	31	17	14,722	1,216
106-115	32	19	24,125	1,623
116-125	33	20	31,665	1,610
126-135	8	21	65,050	3,237
		Mares		
<95	17	18	21,215	1,360
96-105	17	20	13,756	854
106-115	11	19	29,277	1,511
116-125	7	19	29,043	1,552
126-135	1	42	79,120	1,884

**Danish Kroner*

(reprinted from the Equine Veterinary Journal 12 (2) 81-84)

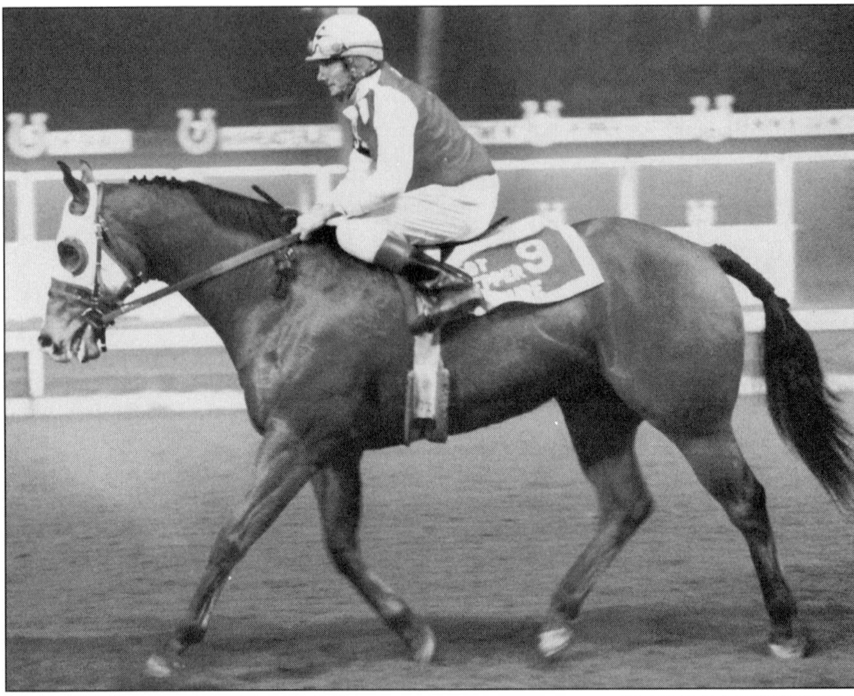

Photo courtesy of the Quarter Horse Racing Journal

Sgt. Pepper Feature

Chapter 19

Quarter Horses Also Have Great Heart

Research has proven that the characteristic in racehorses known as "great heart" is really a physical description of an extraordinary heart found in certain Thoroughbreds, Quarter Horses, Morgans, Saddlebreds, and Standardbreds. From the legendary Eclipse, foaled in England in 1764, this great heart has passed down the female line on the X chromosome.

The heart is also found in Arabians, one of the sources of the great heart introduced into the Thoroughbred in the 1600s. Because Quarter Horses long have been crossed with Thoroughbreds, great Quarter Horse runners can have the same great heart as found in great Thoroughbreds. Today, Eclipse's mighty heart is passed through a number of sires.

The most successful Quarter Horse sires that pass on the large heart have large-hearted Thoroughbred lines on their bottom sides. Thoroughbred heart lines on the top side won't do any good because the characteristic isn't on the Y chromosome, which comes from the sire. In measuring large hearts in different breeds, Dr. Fregin went to the Hall of Champions at the Kentucky Horse Park near Lexington to measure two champions, one a storied Thoroughbred gelding named John Henry and the other a world champion Quarter Horse gelding named Sgt. Pepper Feature.

John Henry is a Horse of the Year with earnings of more than $6.5 million. He was found to have a heart score of 147. Sgt. Pepper Feature is a world champion with earnings of more than $900,000. His heart score was 143. Both of these hearts are extraordinary.

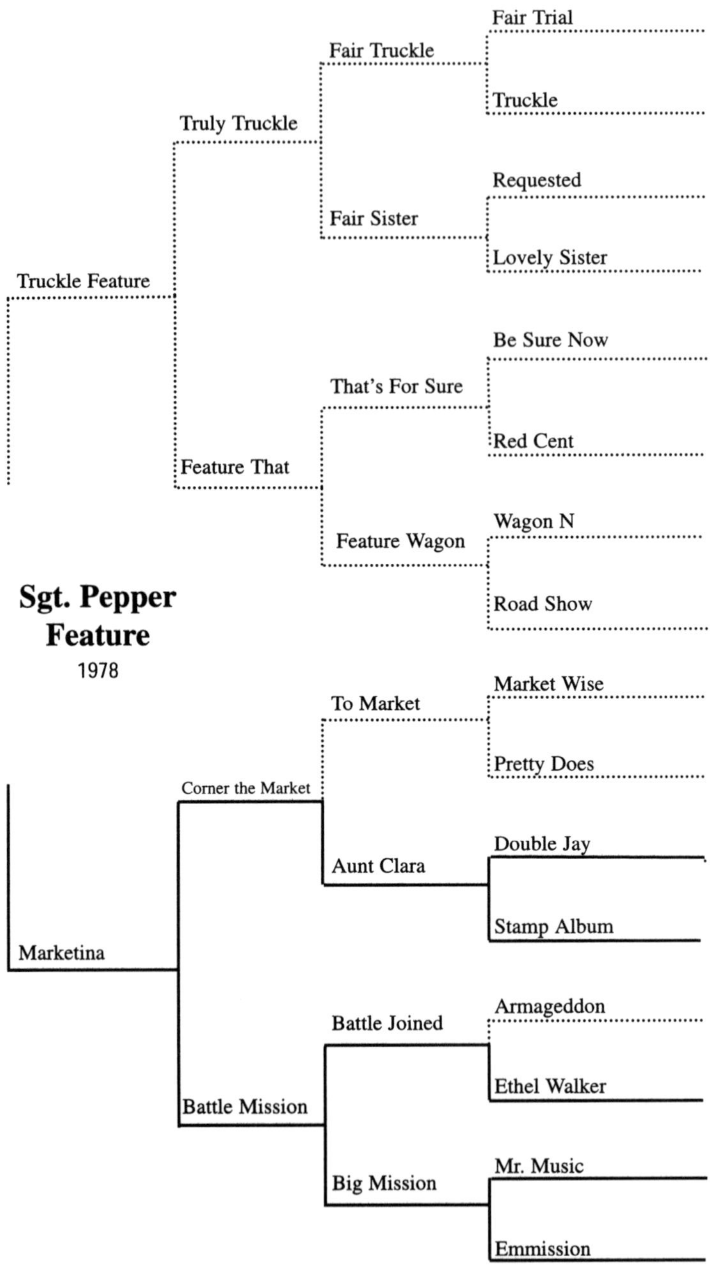
Sgt. Pepper
Feature
1978
Truckle Feature
Truly Truckle
Fair Truckle
Fair Trial
Truckle
Fair Sister
Requested
Lovely Sister
Feature That
That's For Sure
Be Sure Now
Red Cent
Feature Wagon
Wagon N
Road Show
Marketina
Corner the Market
To Market
Market Wise
Pretty Does
Aunt Clara
Double Jay
Stamp Album
Battle Mission
Battle Joined
Armageddon
Ethel Walker
Big Mission
Mr. Music
Emmission

Based on the Australian study comparing heart score to heart weight at autopsy, these horses each have hearts that weigh between 14 and 15 pounds — larger than that of Eclipse. Both horses traced back to the same heart line, that of the great Double Jay (TB). ECG tracings indicated other similarities in heart-rate patterns, adding to the possibility that both geldings carry the same heart.

Double Jay is unique for the large-heart line because he goes to Eclipse both through Pocahontas and through Lexington through the female side of Audience, the dam of his broodmare sire Whisk Broom II. Audience's dam Sallie McClelland is a daughter of the great Hindoo, who was out of the Lexington mare Florence. Sallie McClelland's dam Red and Blue was by Alarm, who was out of Maud, a daughter of Pocahontas's son Stockwell.

When I studied the pedigrees of leading Quarter Horse runners, I found it ironic to see a pattern that has haunted the large-hearted individual for centuries. A Thoroughbred stallion might start his stud career in the rich bluegrass of Kentucky, but when he cannot duplicate himself through a son — an impossibility for the large-heart inheritance — then the spotlight is quickly turned off and he finds himself sent away, frequently to Texas or elsewhere throughout the West and Southwest. Then that great heart, which Kentucky breeders couldn't wait for, often finds its way into the best Quarter Horses, lengthening their distances and increasing their stamina and speed with superior cardiovascular systems.

Chapter 20

Differences in Heart Expression

An interesting observation has been made in measuring racing Quarter Horses as compared with Thoroughbreds. During the formative years of a horse's growth, particularly the first three years, heart size can be increased through conditioning. A small heart can't become a large one but it can be possible to add up to 10 points through training, particularly aerobic training.

This is where we see the difference between the growth of the same heart in a Quarter Horse vs. a Thoroughbred. Quarter Horse trainers don't run their horses in training as often as Thoroughbred trainers. Many like to use the "rubber band" method, meaning they like to wind up the horse before a race and save his running for during the race.

Because the Quarter Horse doesn't get as much aerobic conditioning during training, such as daily two-mile gallops, and because they run shorter distances during a race, they don't build up the heart muscle as much as the Thoroughbred, who spends more time on the track during training and runs at longer distances. Because of this, we don't see quite the expression in a Quarter Horse of a specific heart as we do in a Thoroughbred who has spent more miles galloping on the track during his conditioning.

In measuring Quarter Horses, we have found between a five- and 10-point difference in the heart score of the same heart than is found in the mature Thoroughbred. We have found super hearts in the Quarter Horse. Easy Jet seems to have one of the largest. Sgt. Pepper Feature had a heart score of 143 and we have found that same size in an Easy Jet daughter. In a Quarter Horse,

Easy Jet (right)
and
Three Bars

*Photos courtesy of
The Quarter Racing Journal
and the Thoroughbred Times*

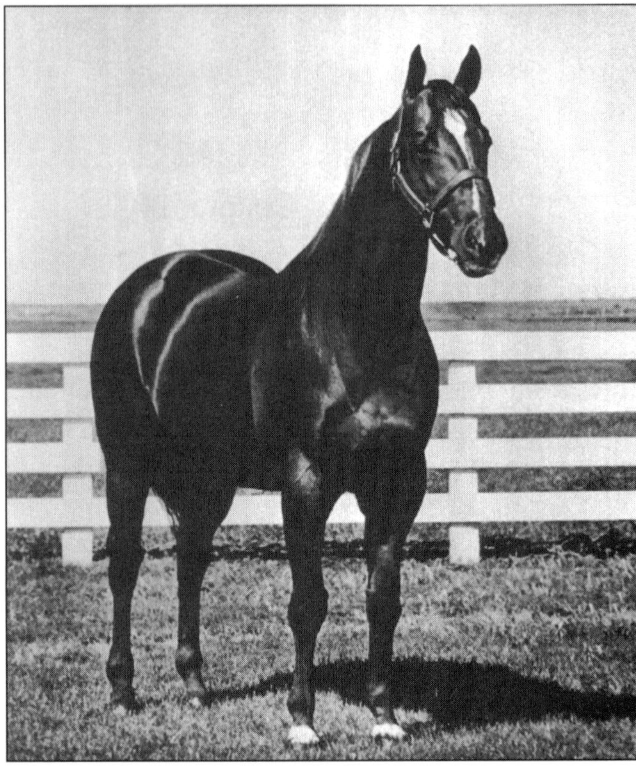

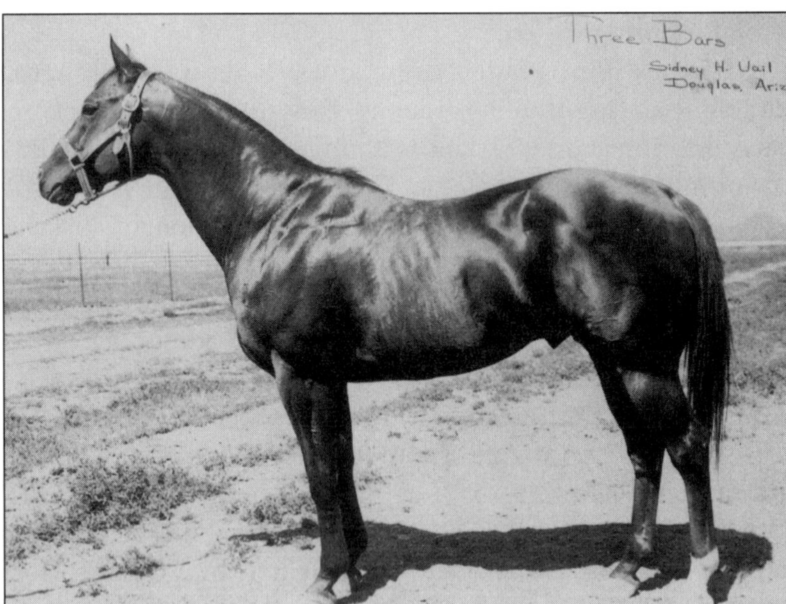

that heart score would be the equivalent of 147-150 in a Thoroughbred. The heart score of Sgt. Pepper Feature, who is out of a Double Jay mare, was close to another Double Jay grandson, the legendary John Henry, who was 147. Reckless Dash, a son of Dash For Cash, carries the heart line of Raise Your Glass (TB), sire of Special Effort. Although his heart lines won't help his sons, on the X chromosome line Raise Your Glass carries the large-heart lines of Bull Lea (TB), Sweep and War Admiral through his dam Champagne Woman.

Streakin Six is another sire with good heart lines. His broodmare sire Little Request (TB) is a maternal grandson of Sweep. While the bottom of his dam's pedigree is pretty good, based on his pattern of performance it is probable that Streakin Six is carrying the Sweep heart.

Carrying the Eclipse heart is champion Ronas Ryon. His dam Rona Bar goes to Eclipse through her sire Three Bargains, who tracks to Lexington twice through his maternal granddam Marina.

In scientific studies of trotters conducted in Denmark by Nielsen and Vibe-Petersen, a positive correlation was shown between earnings and high heart scores. In the study, the 41 stallions with heart scores above 115 earned more than double what the 81 stallions with heart scores below 115 earned.

However, one interesting fact found in the University of Kentucky study is that the size of the horse doesn't seem to have any relation to the size of the heart. The largest hearts aren't necessarily found in the largest horses. While all large hearts track to Eclipse, some lines, whether from genetic modifiers, natural selection or pattern of breeding, have even larger expressions of the large heart found in Eclipse.

Three Bars

1940

- Percentage
  - Midway
    - Ballot
      - Voter
        - Friar's Balsam
        - Mavourneen
      - Cerito
        - Lowland Chief
        - Merry Dance
    - Thirty-Third
      - Sir Dixon
        - Billet
        - Jaconet
      - High Degree
        - His Highness
        - Nettie
  - Gossip Avenue
    - Bulse
      - Disguise II
        - Domino
        - Bonnie Gal
      - Nethersole
        - Tournament
        - Fairy Slipper
    - Rosewood
      - Magneto
        - Star Shoot
        - Marie Frances
      - Rose Tree
        - Bonna Vista
        - Fanny Relph
- Myrtle Dee
  - Luke McLuke
    - Ultimus
      - Commando
        - Domino
        - Emma C
      - Running Stream
        - Domino
        - Dancing Water
    - Midge
      - Trenton
        - Musket
        - Frailty
      - Sandfly
        - Isonomy
        - Sandiway
  - Civil Maid
    - Patriot
      - Ben Brush
        - Bramble
        - Roseville
      - Sandfly
        - Isonomy
        - Sandiway
    - Civil Rule
      - Carlsbad
        - Glenelg
        - Lady Wayward
      - Semper Victoire
        - Logic
        - La Sylphide

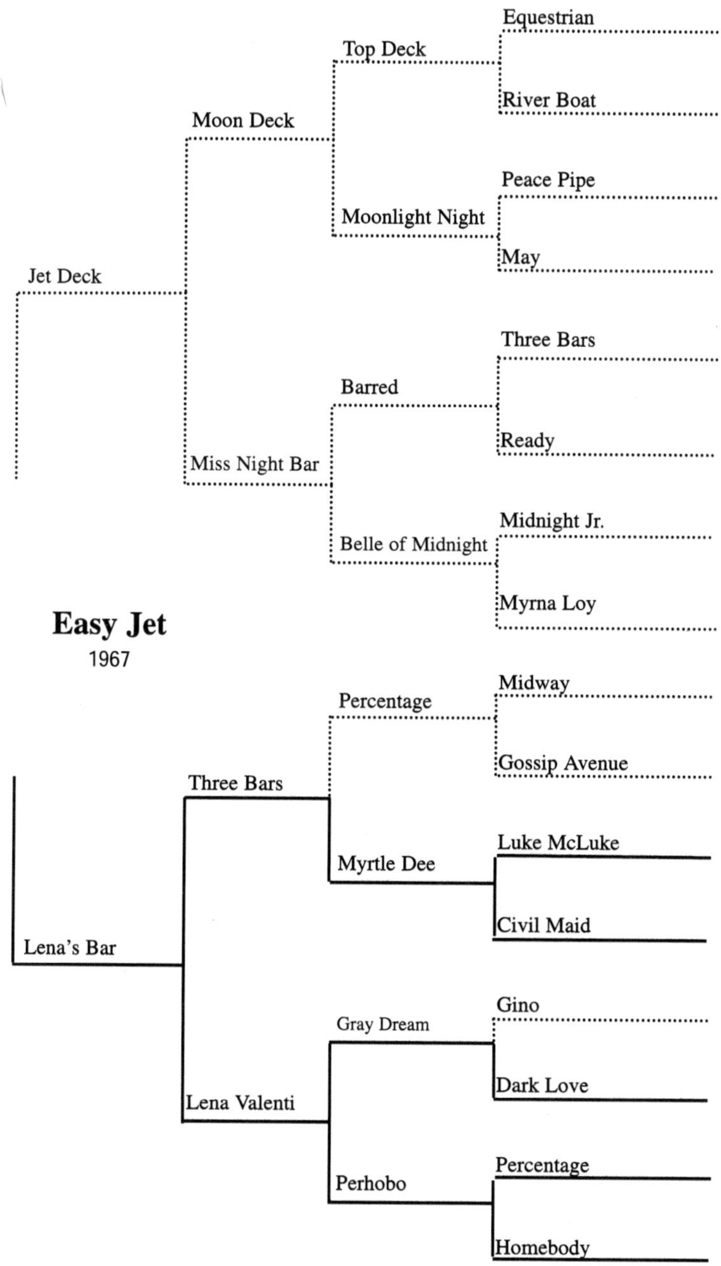
Easy Jet
1967
Jet Deck
Moon Deck
Top Deck
Equestrian
River Boat
Moonlight Night
Peace Pipe
May
Miss Night Bar
Barred
Three Bars
Ready
Belle of Midnight
Midnight Jr.
Myrna Loy
Lena's Bar
Three Bars
Percentage
Midway
Gossip Avenue
Myrtle Dee
Luke McLuke
Civil Maid
Lena Valenti
Gray Dream
Gino
Dark Love
Perhobo
Percentage
Homebody

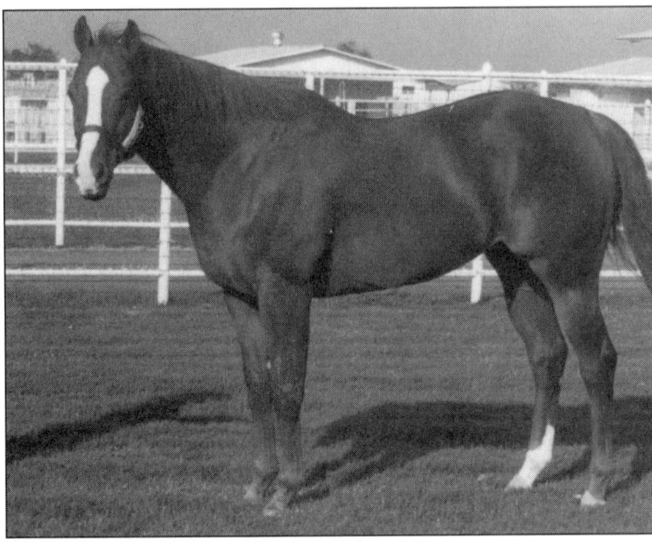

Photo courtesy of Jim Jennings

Dash For Cash

Chapter 21

Dash For Cash

Judging by the pattern of performance in Quarter Horses with large hearts, the high-performance cardiovascular system is just as important in an animal that reaches his sprinting speed in three strides and never lets up until the finish line.

The most successful Quarter Horse sires that pass on the large heart have large-hearted Thoroughbred lines on their bottom sides. Thoroughbred heart lines on the top side won't do any good because the characteristic isn't on the Y chromosome, which comes from the sire.

A prime example of a Quarter Horse with the large Eclipse heart is Dash For Cash. His dam Find A Buyer (TB) goes to the Eclipse heart on the X chromosome through Whirlaway on the tail-female line through his maternal great-granddam Scattered and through his maternal granddam Hide and Seek, a daughter of Alibhai. An outstanding broodmare sire, Alibhai was found to have a 14-pound heart at autopsy.

The Dash For Cash heart is in the 130s. For a Quarter Horse, a 130 heart is considered a super heart. One of his sons, the amazingly successful sire First Down Dash, was found to have such a heart. Rare Form and Pure D Dash also have that heart score. With all three sires one finds very good daughters which will end up being very good producers.

All of Dash For Cash's maternal X chromosome lines go to the Eclipse heart line, but the stallion's success and the success of his daughters on the racetrack suggest that the heart probably comes from either Whirlaway or Alibhai. Following the pattern of other successful large-hearted racehorses, most of the big earners by Dash For Cash were female because they were the only ones able to inherit his heart. All of Dash For Cash's daughters will carry

Dash For Cash

1973

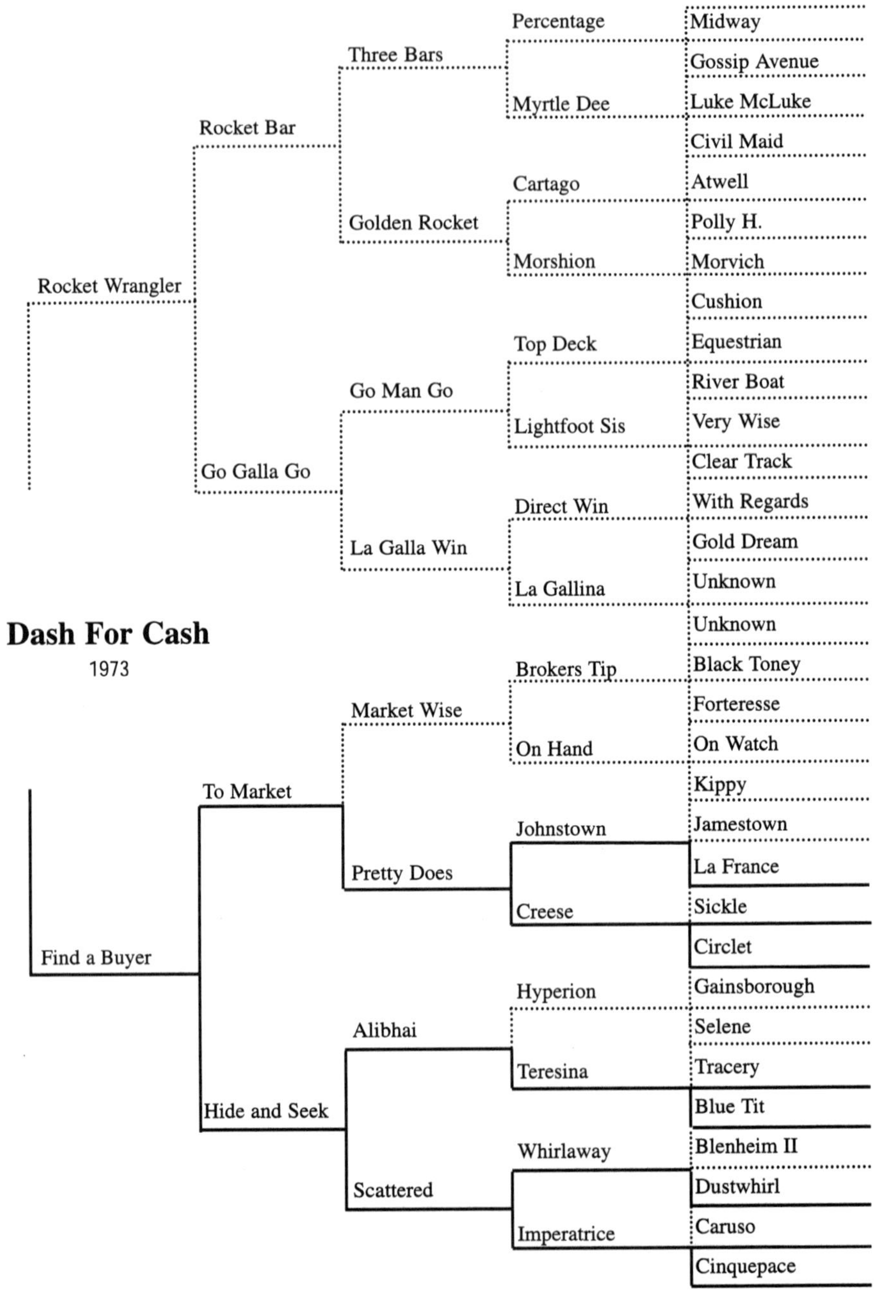

his large-hearted X chromosome. Some will express it and some will carry it as a recessive and be able to give it to half of their offspring. A double-copy daughter would have Dash For Cash on one X and another large-heart on her other X.

In studying the pedigrees of the stallion's best sons, you will find large-heart lines in the pedigrees of their dams. In First Down Dash's case, for example, the large heart comes from his broodmare sire Gallant Jet, who goes to Eclipse through his second dam Linda Jewel, a daughter of Red Jewel (TB) who goes to Eclipse through Pocahontas on all of his female lines. First Down Dash is known both for his sons and his daughters, just like his sire. He's following in his daddy's footsteps in producing outstanding daughters, such as champions Dashing Folly, Ah Sigh, Corona Cash, Corona Kool, Down With Debt, Royal Down Dash and Speedy Empress, all of whom have good bottom sides and should be good producers.

First Down Dash's heart score of 130 is considered very large for a Quarter Horse. He combines the quality of speed and heart which is found in the best sires. This enables him to give speed to both his sons and daughters and a large heart to his daughters. When bred to large-hearted mares, his sons combine the two qualities as well.

Most of those mares have also had outstanding large-heart lines. Champion Dash Thru Traffic is out of Lady Meter Reader, a daughter of large-hearted sire Beduino (TB), whose dam Jo-Ann-Cat was a double-copy daughter of Rejected out of the Depth Charge mare Quick Eye. Lady Meter Reader also is out of a daughter of Tiny Charger. Dash Thru Traffic's maternal great-granddam Rhoda Watch is a daughter of Anchor Watch (TB), who carries the Sweep heart line.

The best producers of a large-hearted sire are frequently double-copy mares. Dash For Cash's champion daughter Florentine is a good example. She earned more than $1.1 million and is out of a double-copy mare, Trippy Dip (TB), who has large-heart lines on all of her X chromosome lines. Trippy Dip is by Scout Leader, who is out of a probable double-copy mare, Polylady, who is by the large-hearted sire Polynesian and out of Lady Dorimar, a granddaughter of Man 'o War.

Trippy Dip's heart lines on her dam's side are even better. Her dam Dancing Straw is by Dancing Dervish who is out of Mumtaz, a daughter of Mahmoud — one of the four largest heart lines. Her maternal granddam is the great Jackstraw mare M. Straw, who demonstrated the pattern of performance and durability found with a superior cardiovascular system when she won a stakes at Ruidoso Downs on Sept. 8, 1963. Twelve days later in Albuquerque, she won a six-furlong race then was hauled 900 miles to New Braunfels, Texas, where on Sept. 28 she ran the fastest three-eighths of a mile recorded in the state.

Jackstraw carried the large-heart lines to Eclipse through his dam Absurdity. Through her dam Inquiry, all roads led to Pocahontas through her sons Stockwell and Rataplan.

Jackstraw also demonstrated the pattern of producing outstanding daughters, including Sea Nymph, his leading earner, and multiple champion Straw Flight. His other accomplished daughters include Fly Straw, Nosey Josey (TB), Kaystorm, Maggie Straw, Cindy Straw, Straw Doll, Straw Lil and Miss Straw. They passed on Jackstraw's great heart to future generations. Because of Trippy Dip's heart line, her champion son Calyx should sire nice daughters and sons when bred to large-hearted mares.

Trippy Dip's rise from the Santa Anita claiming ranks to blue-hen Quarter Horse producer is a good example of the fact that no matter how poorly the world might treat you, you can't keep good genes down. Luckily for the Quarter Horse breed, Trippy Dip's worth was realized and she was crossed with the large-hearted sire Dash For Cash. The rest is history.

One daughter of Dash For Cash that is probably a double-copy mare is Miss Eye Opener, because she has produced six winners from eight starters and one stakes winner, world champion Special Leader. She carries the large heart of Dash For Cash and is out of a daughter of the large-hearted sire Beduino (TB), who has an outstanding bottom side for the large heart. Her second dam Ought To Go is a daughter of the terrific large-hearted sire Go Man Go and is out of a daughter of War Bam, who goes to the large

Sweep heart.

As a result, Special Leader is a sire whose daughters should be worth watching as racehorses and broodmares. Dash For Cash's daughter Flow of Cash was a double-copy mare out of Cherry Lake (TB), another double-copy mare who produced four champions when bred to Dash For Cash. Although she only produced two foals before her death, Flow of Cash, a stakes winner of more than $324,246, did produce a stakes winner in her son Frisco Flare.

Cherry Lake produced six winners from eight starters that earned more than $1.8 million. Following the pattern of double-copy daughters from double-copy dams, Cherry Lake's daughter Rain Onya (by Go Man Go) produced double-copy Shake It to Em, by Dash For Cash. Shake It to Em continued the pattern, producing eight winners from nine starters with two stakes winners. When champion Elan Again was bred to Dash For Cash, she produced the filly Dash Again, an earner of $254,068 who has produced seven winners from eight starters, with three stakes winners and the earners of more than $1.5 million. Dash Again followed her double-copy dam's pattern when she was bred to Special Effort and produced the double-copy filly Elans Special, who won the All American Futurity (G1).

Champion Corona Chick is a double-copy mare. She carries the large-hearted X from her sire Chicks Beduino, who goes to Eclipse through his maternal granddam Mayshego. On her bottom side, through her dam Sizzling Lil, Corona Cash has heart lines through Leo and the super heart of Blue Larkspur (TB) through her tail-female line. Corona Chick's daughter champion Corona Cash also will be a double-copy mare because she is by the large-hearted sire First Down Dash. Corona Cash should prove to be a good producer like her dam.

We measured Corona Cutie, who is out of Corona Chick's full-sister Corona Wild, and found a very large heart. Measured at two, Corona Cutie already had a heart score of 133+ with the possibility of maturing to 140+, a very large heart for a Quarter Horse. We also measured champion Corona Kool, who at three had a heart score of 130+. She is a prime example of a "liberated filly"

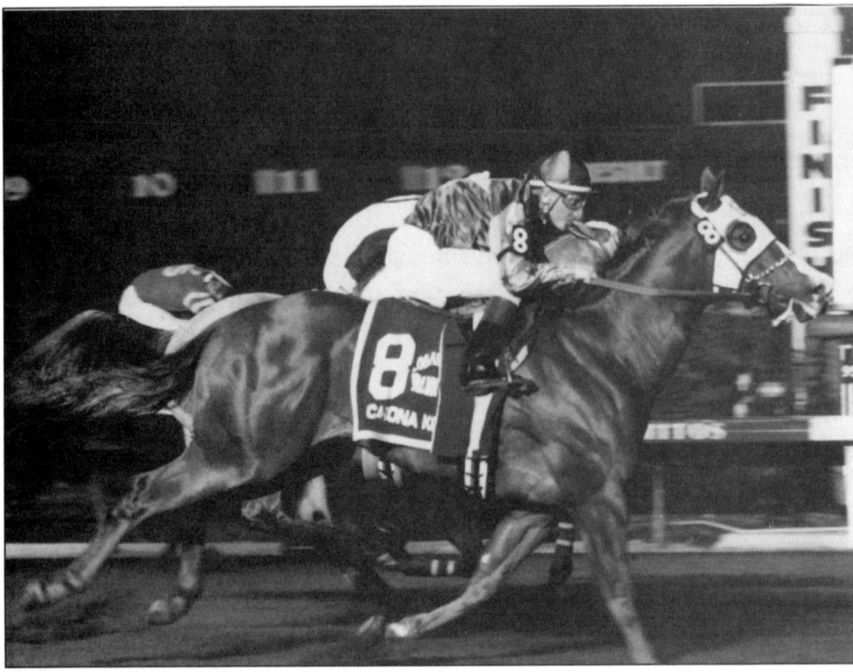

Photo by Scott Martinez; courtesy of the American Quarter Horse Journal

Corona Kool (First Down Dash x Sizzling Lil)

who produces babies while she keeps up her career as a successful racehorse.

After a nine-month layoff, the 1999 champion two-year-old filly came back to the races at four and won the California Breeders Matron Stakes (RG3) by 2 3/4 lengths to boost her bankroll to more than $1million while somebody else raised the babies. In 2001 she had a weanling by Chick's Beduino on the ground while a surrogate mare incubates her 2002 foal by Devon Lane, a Thoroughbred son of Storm Cat. Both Corona Cutie and Corona Kool were by First Down Dash, whose heart score is 130. Corona Kool probably carries her sire's heart and Corona Cutie probably gets her large heart from her granddam Sizzling Lil, the dam of Corona Kool.

In Sizzling Lil's pedigree, her second dam Here's To Lil is a daughter of the Thoroughbred Exalted Rullah. Exalted Rullah's dam Echoic is by All Blue, who is out of Blue Delight, a daughter of Blue Larkspur, one of the four major super hearts in the modern

Corona Kool

1997

- First Down Dash
  - Dash for Cash
    - Rocket Wrangler
      - Rocket Bar
      - Go Galla Go
    - Find a Buyer
      - To Market
      - Hide And Seek
  - First Prize Rose
    - Gallant Jet
      - Jet Deck
      - Leo Jewel
    - Rose Bug
      - Lady Bug's Moon
      - Casco Rose
- Sizzling Lil
  - Sizzle Te
    - Azure Te
      - Nashville
      - Blue One
    - Jet's Fair Lady
      - Jet Deck
      - Sooner Lady
  - Lilsalady
    - Reb's Policy
      - New Policy
      - Yenoh Reb
    - Here's To Lil
      - Exalted Rullah
      - Jumpin Jackie

Thoroughbred. A 140+ heart score is in keeping with this heartline.

Because these two fillies carry their sire's X with a 130 heart score and their dam's X with a 140+ heart score, they should be able to produce superior hearts in all of their offspring when mated to large-hearted sires. All of their daughters should also make superior double-copy mares. Corona Cartel, Corona Chick's son who earned $557,142 before entering stud this year, also should have a large heart. His daughters should be outstanding, and his sons — if he is bred to large-hearted mares — also should find the winner's circle.

Remember, the best-producing daughters are not always the best racers, which is true in all breeds. There are many different reasons why some individuals don't make it on the track, such as finances, injury or poor training. But they still can carry the genes of champions and can produce. Two examples of Dash For Cash mares that fit this category are Cypress Point, who never raced but produced three winners from three starters, including champion Develop A Plan and the earners of more than $390,000; and Cash Balance, dam of stakes winners Six Figures, Fabulous Figure and Six On the Beach, who earned only $425 on the track but has produced six winners from seven starters with earnings of more than $465,000.

Six On the Beach is a probable double copy with large-heart lines on all of her pedigree lines. Merry For Cash, with a 106 speed index, is another example of a good producing daughter by Dash For Cash. She has seven winners from eight starters and three stakes winners. She probably received the Depth Charge (TB) heart from her broodmare sire Midway Mayor (TB).

Especially For You is an example of a probable single copy. She didn't express Dash For Cash's heart, but had it to give to champion Rare Form, who now can pass it on to his daughters such as champion Fabulous Form. He also will sire winning sons like champion Especially Rare when he is bred to mares like Me Bright Special, daughter of large-hearted sire Special Effort.

Rare Form's heart score was measured at 130, which we also found in two of his daughters. He looks very much like Dash

For Cash, so it is assumed he is passing Dash For Cash's heart. Dashing Phoebe not only expressed Dash For Cash's heart and earned $609,554, but when bred to Special Effort she produced champion Special Phoebe.

Darlin Dash might not have expressed her sire's heart, but she produced champion Darlin Sixarun. Millionaire Make Mine Cash expressed her sire's heart and produced champion Make Mine Bud. Make Mine Cash has some holes in the bottom side of her pedigree, which might explain her produce record of 10 foals with eight starters, four winners and one stakes winner.

Dash For Speed earned more than $1.2 million but hasn't produced up to her potential. She has some genetic holes in her bottom side for the large heart and is a probable single copy, so she should always should be bred to a large-hearted sire — while a prayer is said for the correct X to come up in the mix. Daughters of Dash For Speed, such as the two she has by Special Effort, eventually might produce large-hearted individuals. Even if they received the wrong X from Dash For Speed, they will carry the large heart of their sire.

Like all great sires, Dash for Cash has been successful with both genders. One of his greatest sons, First Down Dash, who received a large heart from his dam, has been an extraordinary sire. He is also known for both his sons and his daughters.

First Down Dash combines the quality of speed and heart which is found in the best sires. This enables him to give speed to both his sons and daughters and a large heart to his daughters. When bred to large-hearted mares, his sons combine the two qualities as well.

We measured a daughter of First Down Dash, First Down 'n Surfin, who finished third in the All American Futurity in 2000 while still a maiden. A daughter of In the Curl, a Thoroughbred mare by Shelter Half, who is out of a daughter of Sir Gaylord (half-brother to Secretariat), First Down 'n Surfin might end up with Sir Gaylord's heart which would give her First Down Dash's great heart on one X and Sir Gaylord's on the other X. When she was measured at two, before the All American Futurity, she already had a larger heart than her dam, a speed ball that had earned more than $769,000 racing for Secretariat's owner Penny Chenery.

First Down 'n Surfin was already approaching the heart score of her sire with two more years to grow, so it seemed conceivable that she would end up with Sir Gaylord's heart. When she goes to the breeding shed she should be a terrific producer.

From the other gender comes First Down Dash's son, champion Royal Quick Dash. He is out of a Beduino mare, Harems Choice, who is out of a daughter of Tiny Charger. His maternal great-granddam Hy Flicka is a daughter of Hysition (TB), who traces back to Eclipse through Pocahontas.

A Classic Dash, another champion son of First Down Dash, also comes from a dam with good heart lines. Classic Canyon (TB) is a daughter of Dusty Canyon, who goes to Eclipse through his broodmare sire Goya II. A Classic Dash's second dam Like Grandma is a daughter of David Cox, who is out of the great Three Bars mare Miss Myrna Bar. Three Bars brought into the Quarter Horse breed one of its largest hearts. His dam Myrtle Dee goes to Eclipse both through her sire and her dam. Her sire Luke McLuke goes to Pocahontas' great son Stockwell through Isonomy. Her dam Civil Maid goes to Isonomy through her broodmare sire, Patriot, and her second dam Civil Rule goes to Eclipse through her sire Carlsbad, whose second dam traces back to Eclipse as well.

Three Bars is the large heart influence in one of the largest hearts found so far in our measurements of Quarter Horses - Easy Jet. With a heart score of 143+ based on measurements of his daughters, Easy Jet was able to do phenomenal things on the track. So did some of his daughters, which have also been very good producers, especially when bred to large-hearted sires like Dash For Cash. Grade 1 winner Holland Ease, a son of First Down Dash who earned a 109 speed index, carries plenty of heart through his dam Easy Henryetta, a daughter of Easy Jet. Easy Henryetta's second dam Baby Steel (TB) is by Leadstealer, who is out of a daughter of the influential Mahmoud. Easy Henryetta has been measured and found to have a very large heart.

First Down Dash

1984

- Dash for Cash
  - Rocket Wrangler
    - Rocket Bar
      - Three Bars
      - Golden Rocket
    - Go Galla Go
      - Go Man Go
      - La Galla Win
  - Find a Buyer
    - To Market
      - Market Wise
      - Pretty Does
    - Hide and Seek
      - Alibhai
      - Scattered
- First Prize Rose
  - Gallant Jet
    - Jet Deck
      - Moon Deck
      - Miss Night Bar
    - Leo Jewel
      - Leo
      - Linda Jewel
  - Rose Bug
    - Lady Bug's Moon
      - Top Moon
      - FL Lady Bug
    - Casco Rose
      - Levan
      - Prissy Hankins

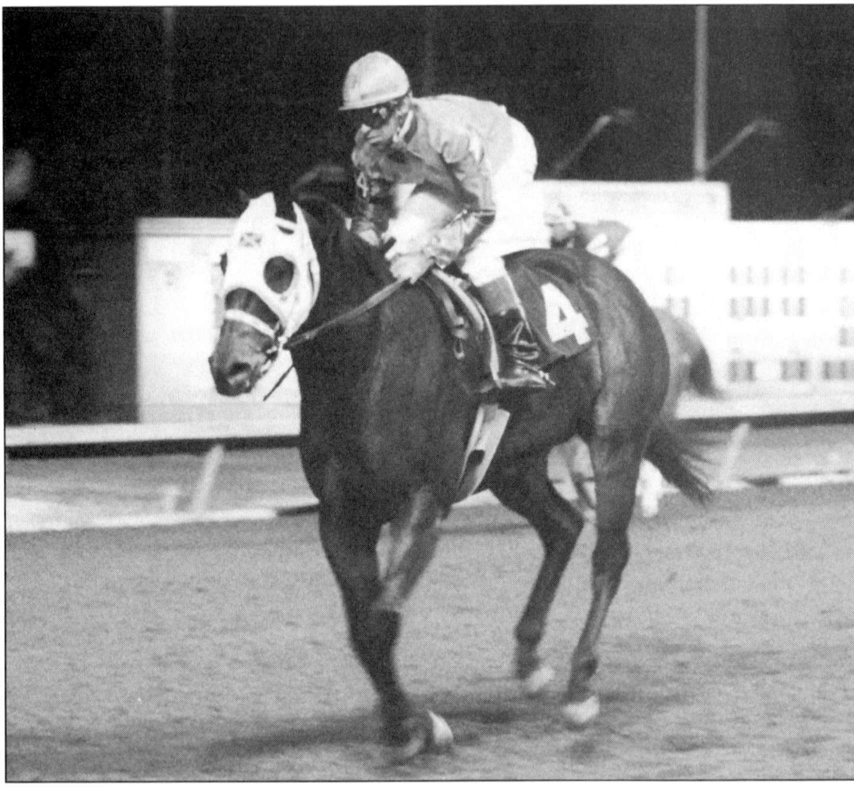

Photo courtesy of the Quarter Horse Racing Journal

Florentine

Florentine

1984

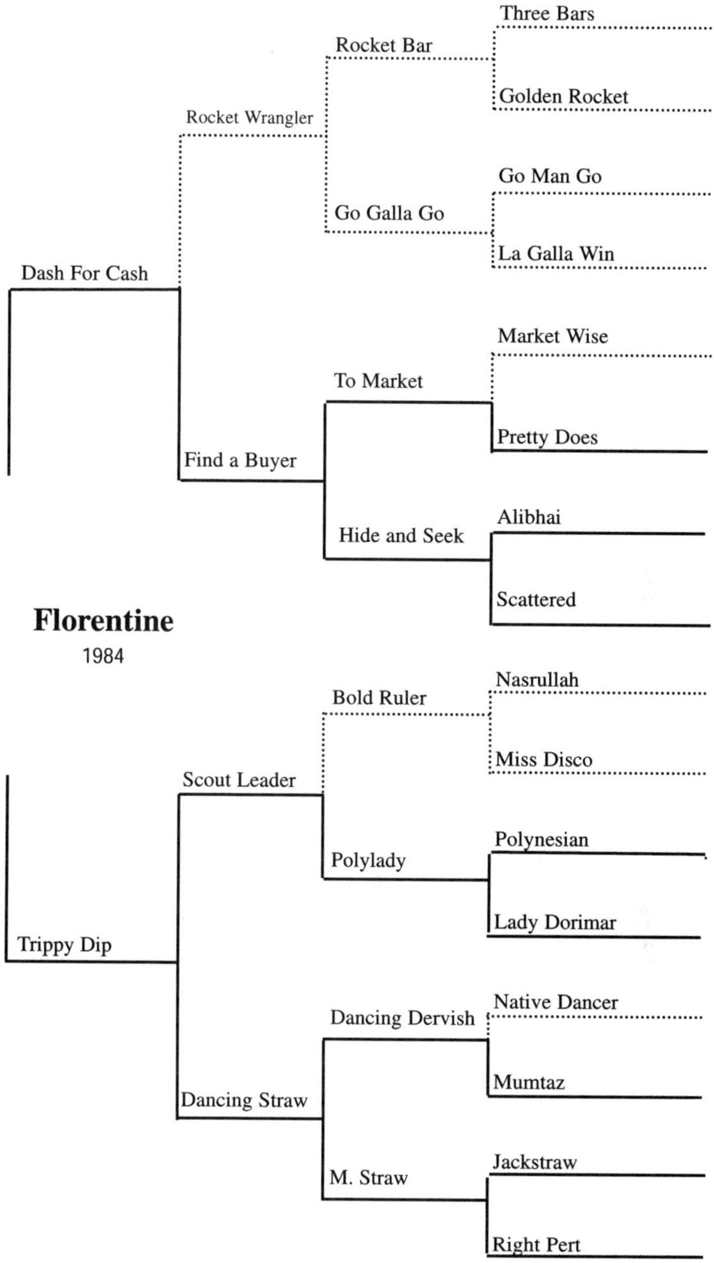

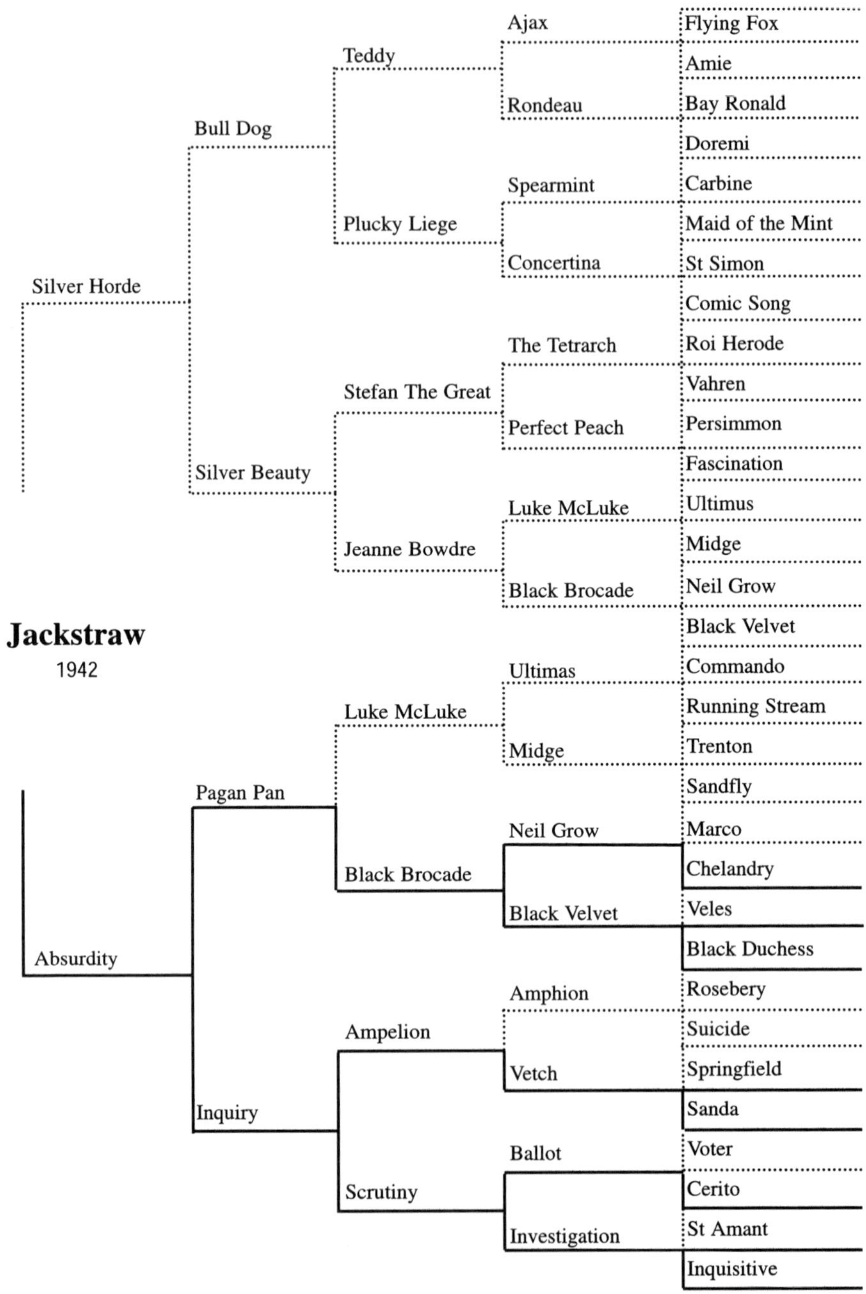
Jackstraw
1942
Silver Horde
Bull Dog
Teddy
Ajax
Flying Fox
Amie
Rondeau
Bay Ronald
Doremi
Plucky Liege
Spearmint
Carbine
Maid of the Mint
Concertina
St Simon
Comic Song
Silver Beauty
Stefan The Great
The Tetrarch
Roi Herode
Vahren
Perfect Peach
Persimmon
Fascination
Jeanne Bowdre
Luke McLuke
Ultimus
Midge
Black Brocade
Neil Grow
Black Velvet
Absurdity
Pagan Pan
Luke McLuke
Ultimas
Commando
Running Stream
Midge
Trenton
Sandfly
Black Brocade
Neil Grow
Marco
Chelandry
Black Velvet
Veles
Black Duchess
Inquiry
Ampelion
Amphion
Rosebery
Suicide
Vetch
Springfield
Sanda
Scrutiny
Ballot
Voter
Cerito
Investigation
St Amant
Inquisitive

Because Quarter Horses long have been crossed with Thoroughbreds, the great heart line found its way into the sprinters years before AQHA was established. This list is an example of some of the large-hearted horses out there today. Sires carrying Eclipse's mighty heart on their X line include:

A Classic Dash
Aforethought (TB)
Alamitos Bar
Ausual Suspect
Azure Te (TB)
Beduino (TB)
Bugs Alive In 75
Bully Bullion
Calyx
Chasin Women
Chicaro Bill
Chicks Beduino
Corona Cartel
Corona Cocktail
Dash For Cash
Dash Thru Traffic
Dashing La Jolla
David Cox
Depth Charge (TB)
Diamond Charge
Dividend
Double Devil
Easy Jet
Especially Rare
Eyesa Special
Feature Mr. Jess
First Down Dash
First Illusions
First Smart Money
Go Man Go
Hempen (TB)
Heza Fast Man
Holland Ease
Jackstraw (TB)
Jet Smooth
Jonny Apollo
Lake Erie (TB)
Leaving Memories
Leo
Little Request (TB)
Merridoc
Mr. Eye Opener
Mr. Jess Perry
Mito Paint (TB)
Moolah Bux (TB)
Moon Deck
Moving Effort
On A High
Pass 'Em Up (TB)
Piggin String (TB)
Pure D Dash
Raise Your Glass (TB)
Rare Bar
Rare Form
Reckless Dash
Rocket Wrangler
Ronas Ryon
Royal Quick Dash
Special Effort
Special Leader
Spotted Bull (TB)
Stoli
Strawfly Special
Streakin La Jolla
Streakin Six
Takin On The Cash
Texas Dancer (TB)
The Signature
This Snow is Royal
Three Bargains
Three Bars (TB)
Three Chicks
Three Oh's
Tiny Charger
Top Deck (TB)

Man 'o War

1917

Fair Play	Hastings	Spendthrift	Australian	West Australian
				Emilia
			Aerolite	Lexington
				Florine
		Cinderella	Tomahawk	King Tom
				Mincemeat
			Manna	Brown Bread
				Tartlet
	Fairy Gold	Bend Or	Doncaster	Stockwell
				Marigold
			Rouge Rose	Thormanby
				Ellen Horne
		Dame Masham	Galliard	Galopin
				Mavis
			Pauline	Hermit
				Lady Masham
Mahubah	Rock Sand	Sainfoin	Springfield	St. Albans
				Viridis
			Sanda	Wenlock
				Sandal
		Roquebrune	St. Simon	Galopin
				St. Angela
			St. Marguerite	Hermit
				Devotion
	Merry Token	Merry Hampton	Hampton	Lord Clifden
				Lady Langden
			Doll Tearsheet	Broomielaw
				Mrs. Quickly
		Mizpah	Macgregor	Macaroni
				Necklace
			Mare by Underhand	Underhand
				The Slayer's Dau.

Chapter 22

Man 'o War and the Quarter Horse

In studying the pedigrees of some of the best runners, sires and dams in Quarter Horse racing, I am amazed at the number of great Thoroughbred hearts that are racing in today's Quarter Horse. One of the greatest is Man 'o War. His heart is found in sires such as Spotted Bull (TB), Spy Song (TB) and Moolah Bux (TB). Each stallion was out of a daughter or granddaughter of Man 'o War.

Special Effort is a good example of a Quarter Horse with the Man 'o War heart. His dam Go Effortlessly is a daughter of Double Devil, who is out of a daughter of Spotted Bull. Go Effortlessly is inbred to Man 'o War through her dam Hijo Beauty (TB), another daughter of Spotted Bull.

Special Effort's son Strawfly Special is an example of what can be produced when an outstanding sire is bred to a double-copy mare. His dam Fly In The Pie produced six starters from six foals, with four winners and one stakes winner. She goes to Eclipse through her sire Pie In The Sky, who is out of Miss Jelly Roll, a daughter of Roulade (TB), who carries the Sweep (TB) and Alibhai (TB) heart lines. Her dam Flying Rockette, by Rocket Bar (TB), is out of the great Jackstraw (TB) mare Fly Straw.

The Signature is another sire who carries the Man 'o War heart line, through his broodmare sire Moolah Bux. His second dam Mable Chick carries large-heart lines to Eclipse through her sire Triple Chick and her broodmare sire Wild Chicle (TB). Judging by the pattern of performance through his female line, it is probable that The Signature expresses the Man 'o War heart. Merridoc also carries the Man 'o War heart line through Spy Song, who sired his

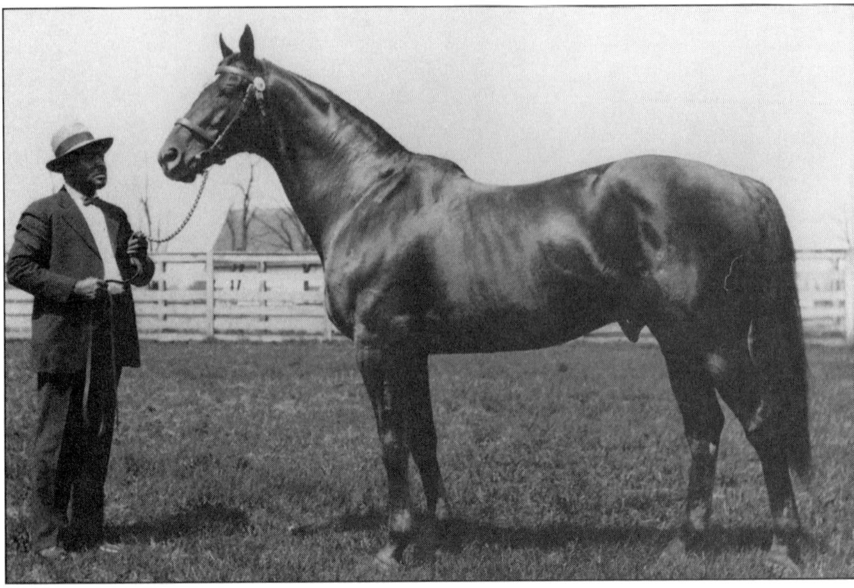

Photos courtesy of the Grayson/Sutcliffe Collection, the Keeneland Library/J.C. Skeets Meadors and Quarter Horse Racing Journal

Conformation photos shown clockwise are Man 'o War (above), Spotted Bull (top right), Hempen (middle right), Spy Song, (bottom right) and Merridoc (below).

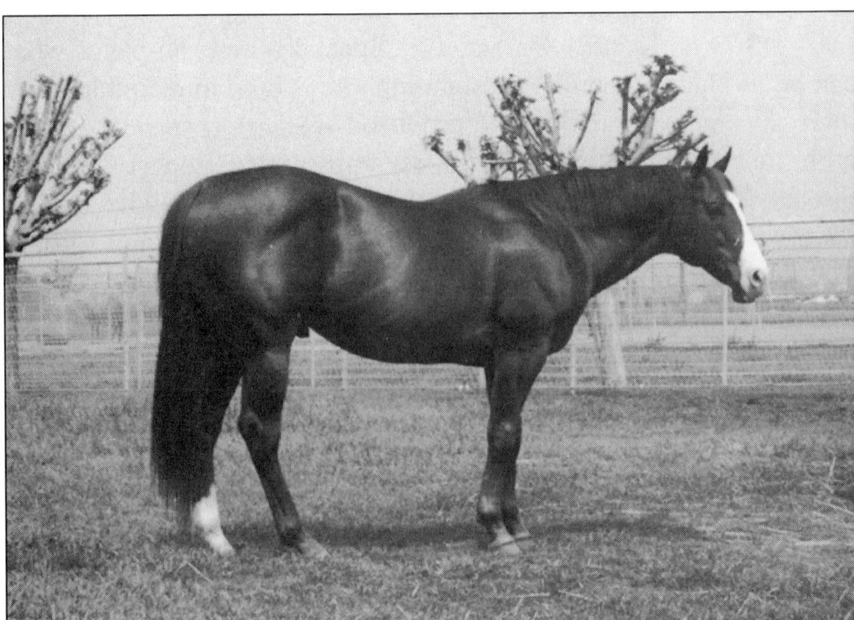

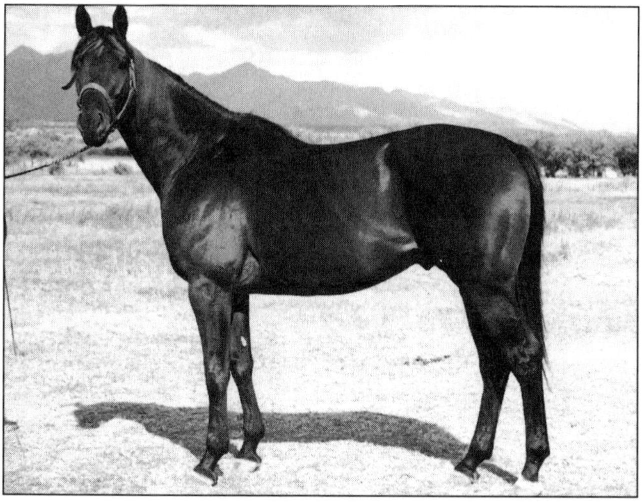

Spotted Bull

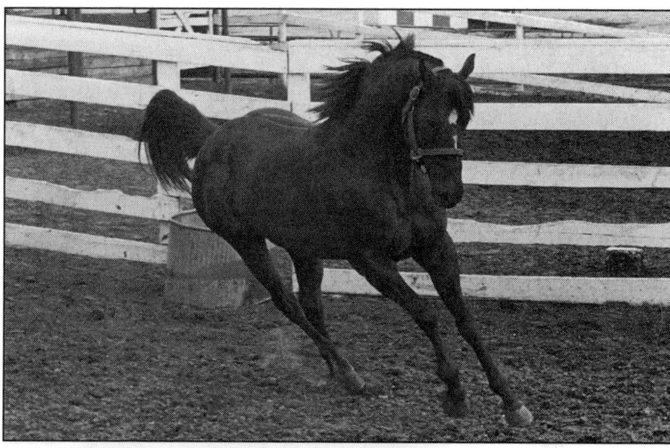

Hempen

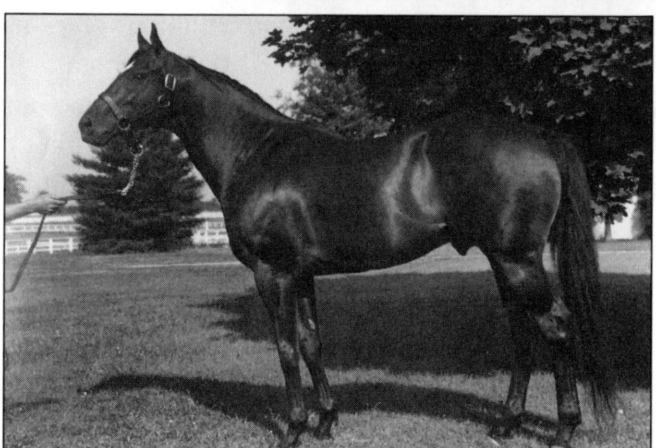

Spy Song

second dam Tiptoe Tune (TB). Merridoc's dam Sparkling Tip is a probable double copy, carrying the Depth Charge (TB) line through her sire Diamond Charge and going to two large-hearted sires on her bottom side, Bolero (TB) and Spy Song.

Following the pattern of large-hearted sires, Merridoc has sired a champion daughter, St. Willa. He is also the broodmare sire of world champion Down With Debt, who, because she is by First Down Dash, could be a double-copy mare. So far, she has produced three starters and two winners.

Another large-hearted sire that has made himself felt on the heart lines of top Quarter Horses is Hempen (TB), who goes to both Man 'o War and his great son War Admiral. Hempen is found on the X chromosome lines of champion Dashing Folly through his daughter Hempes Folly. Another champion by First Down Dash is Speedy Empress, who has Hempen as her maternal great-grandsire. The Hempen heart line can be found in sons of First Down Dash as well. Grade 1 winner Rakin in the Cash, who entered stud this year, is out of a Hempen mare. Leaving Memories is also out of a daughter of Hempen.

One of the things that Man 'o War passed to his descendants along with his great heart is his front end. When comparing the front ends of horses like Spy Song, Mata Hari (his dam), Hempen, Man 'o War's dam, Mahubah, and others you can't help being struck by the physical similarity. Given the soundness of this line, it makes you wonder if there wasn't something about this front end that adapted so well to the type of hard-pounding running seen in Quarter Horse races where they are at top speed from the start. It might help explain why this particular horse has had such an influence in Quarter Horse racing. Whether it was conformation or great heart, Man 'o War had plenty of both to spare. He gave it to both Thoroughbreds and Quarter Horses alike.

Spotted Bull
1946

Bull Dog	Teddy	Ajax	Flying Fox
			Orme
			Vampire
			Amie
			Clamart
			Alice
		Rondeau	Bay Ronald
			Hampton
			Black Duchess
			Doremi
			Bend Or
			Lady Emily
	Plucky Liege	Spearmint	Carbine
			Musket
			The Mersey
			Maid of the Mint
			Minting
			Warble
		Concertina	St. Simon
			Galopin
			St. Angela
			Comic Song
			Petrarch
			Frivolity
Spotted Beauty	Man 'o War	Fair Play	Hastings
			Spendthrift
			Cinderella
			Fairy Gold
			Bend Or
			Dame Masham
		Mahubah	Rock Sand
			Sainfoin
			Roquebrune
			Merry Token
			Merry Hampton
			Mizpah
	Silver Beauty	Stefan The Great	The Tetrarch
			Roi Herode
			Vehren
			Perfect Peach
			Persimmon
			Fascination
		Jeanne Bowdre	Luke McLuke
			Ultimus
			Midge
			Black Brocade
			Neil Gow
			Black Velvet

Spy Song
1943

- Balladier
  - Black Toney
    - Peter Pan
      - Commando
        - Domino
        - Emma C
      - Cinderella
        - Hermit
        - Mazurka
    - Belgravia
      - Ben Brush
        - Bramble
        - Roseville
      - Bonnie Gal
        - Galopin
        - Bonnie Doon
  - Blue Warbler
    - North Star III
      - Sunstar
        - Sundridge
        - Doris
      - Angelic
        - St Angelo
        - Fota
    - May Bird
      - Thrush
        - Missel Thrush
        - Chemistry
      - May Bruce
        - May Duke
        - Lady Bruce
- Mata Hari
  - Peter Hastings
    - Peter Pan
      - Commando
        - Domino
        - Emma C
      - Cinderella
        - Hermit
        - Mazurka
    - Nettie Hastings
      - Hastings
        - Spendthrift
        - Cinderella
      - Princess Nettie
        - His Highness
        - Nettie
  - War Woman
    - Man 'o War
      - Fair Play
        - Hastings
        - Fairy Gold
      - Mahubah
        - Rock Sand
        - Merry Token
    - Topaz
      - Uncle
        - Star Shoot
        - The Niece
      - Ruby Nethersole
        - Star Ruby
        - Nethersole

Hempen
1962

Indian Hemp	Nasrullah	Nearco	Pharos	Phalaris
				Scapa Flow
			Nogara	Havresac II
				Catnip
		Mumtaz Begum	Blenheim II	Blandford
				Malva
			Mumtaz Mahal	The Tetrarch
				Lady Josephine
	Sabzy	Stardust	Hyperion	Gainsborough
				Selene
			Sister Stella	Friar Marcus
				Etoile
		Sarita	Swynford	John O'Gaunt
				Canterbury Pilgrim
			Molly Desmond	Desmond
				Pretty Polly
Serry	Spy Song	Balladier	Black Toney	Peter Pan
				Belgravia
			Blue Warbler	North Star III
				May Bird
		Mata Hari	Peter Hastings	Peter Pan
				Nettie Hastings
			War Woman	Man 'o War
				Topaz
	Santa Roseanna	Rosemont	The Porter	Sweep
				Ballet Girl
			Garden Rose	Colin
				Gardenof Allah
		Sandury	War Admiral	Man O'War
				Brushup
			Minnant	Pennant
				Minaret II

Merridoc

1977

- Tiny's Gay
  - Tiny Watch
    - Anchor Watch
      - Degage
        - Bull Lea
        - Ministress
      - L'Admiralte
        - GrandAdmiral
        - Step Away
    - Clabber Tiny
      - Clabber II
        - Clabber
        - Do Good
      - Tiny Iny
        - Perifox
        - Tiny Rose
  - Gay's Delight
    - Rocket Bar
      - Three Bars
        - Percentage
        - Myrtle Dee
      - Golden Rocket
        - Cartago
        - Morshion
    - Miss Ginger Gay
      - Palleo Pete
        - Leo
        - Osage Star Lady
      - Ginger Gay
        - Bob E
        - Clabber Lady
- Sparkling Tip
  - Diamond Charge
    - Hy Diamond
      - Hygro
        - Epinard
        - Ruddy Light
      - Sirita
        - Jack High
        - Chanciest
    - Lovely Lupita
      - Depth Charge
        - Bold Venture
        - Quickly
      - Dimple McCue
        - Humdinger
        - Lady Vester
  - Tiptoe Tune
    - Spy Song
      - Balladier
        - Black Toney
        - Blue Warbler
      - Mata Hari
        - Peter Hastings
        - War Woman
    - Apoora
      - Bolero
        - Eight Thirty
        - Stepwisely
      - Lazy Me
        - Pavot
        - Sleepytime Gal

The Signature
1980

Parents	Grandparents	Great-grandparents	Great-great-grandparents	Great-great-great-grandparents
Noholme II	Star Kingdom	Stardust	Hyperion	Gainsborough
				Selene
			Sister Stella	Friar Marcus
				Etoile
		Impromptu	Concerto	Orpheus
				Constellation
			Thoughtless	Papyrus
				Virgin's Folly
	Oceana	Colombo	Manna	Phalaris
				Waffles
			Lady Nairne	Chaucer
				Lammermuir
		Orama	Diophon	Grand Parade
				Diadem
			Cantelupe	Amadis
				Lupercalia
Mable Chick Too	Moolah Bux	Mahmoud	Blenheim II	Blandford
				Malva
			Mah Mahal	Gainsborough
				Mumtaz Mahal
		Anchors Ahead	Man 'o War	Fair Play
				Mahubah
			Friar's Carse	Friar Rock
				Problem
	Mable Chick	Triple Chick	Three Bars	Percentage
				Myrtle Dee
			Chicado	Chicaro Bill
				Do Good
		Wild Mable	Wild Chicle	Chicle
				Wild Denise
			Mable Tet	Tetros
				Odd Foot

Special Effort

1979

- Raise Your Glass
  - Raise A Native
    - Native Dancer
      - Polynesian
        - Unbreakable
        - Black Polly
      - Geisha
        - Discovery
        - Miyako
    - Raise You
      - Case Ace
        - Teddy
        - Sweetheart
      - Lady Glory
        - American Flag
        - Beloved
  - Champagne Woman
    - Barbizon
      - Polynesian
        - Unbreakable
        - Black Polly
      - Good Blood
        - Bull Lea
        - Diagnosis
    - L'Amour Toujours
      - Never Say Die
        - Nasrullah
        - Singing Grass
      - Idle Lovliness
        - Casanova
        - The Drone
- Go Effortlessly
  - Double Devil
    - Double Bid
      - Double Feature
        - Psychic Bid
        - Cinema
      - Paula Thomasina
        - Chicaro's Tom
        - Mary Story
    - Bella St Mary
      - Spotted Bull
        - Bull Dog
        - Spotted Beauty
      - Dolly Mack
        - Ace of Diamonds
        - Billie M
  - Hijo Beauty
    - Spotted Bull
      - Bull Dog
        - Teddy
        - Plucky Liege
      - Spotted Beauty
        - Man O'War
        - Silver Beauty
    - Hijo Lanty
      - Hijo Manso
        - Hijo Mio
        - Manceba
      - Sky Lanty
        - Sir Lanny
        - Pretty Pol

Anchor Watch

1953

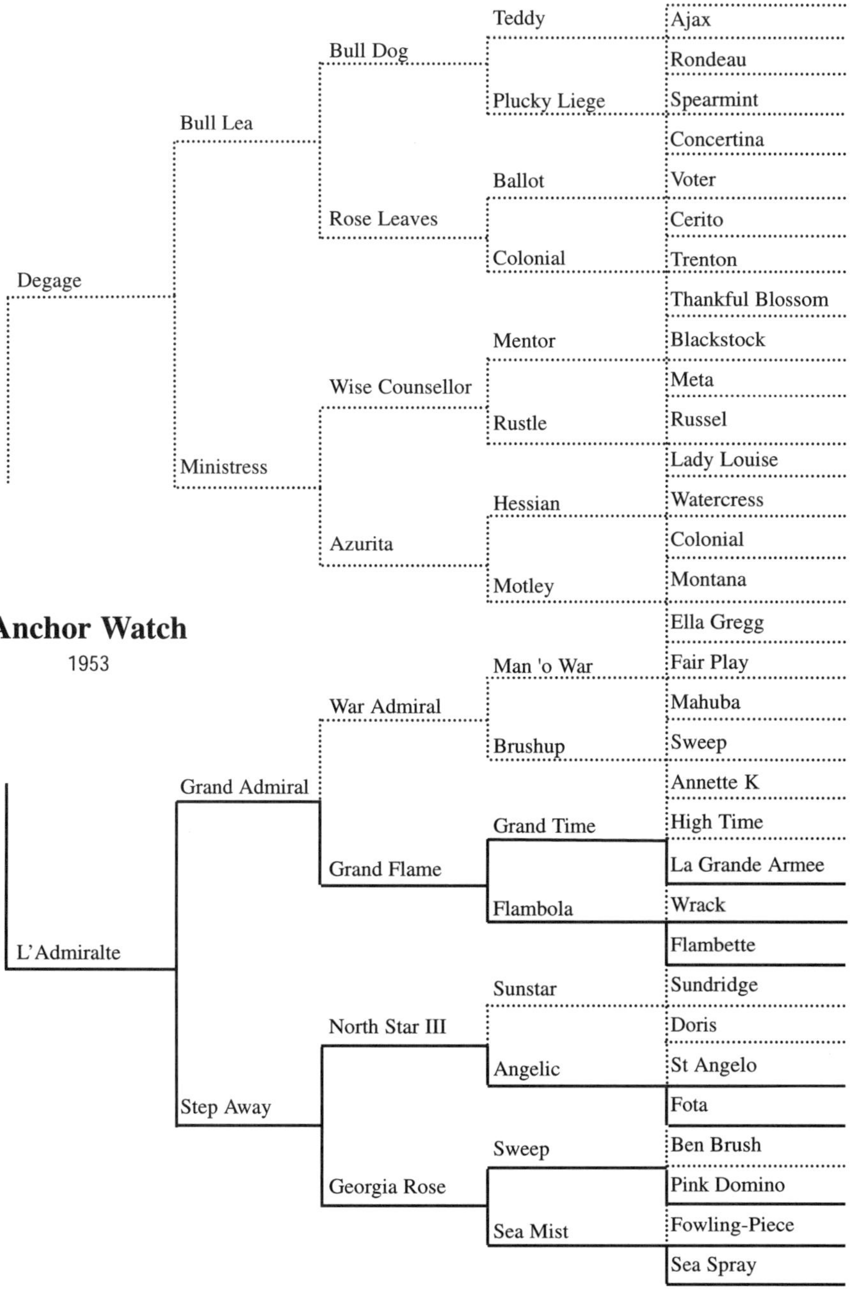

Chapter 23

Great Hearts and Their ECGs

In the past six years, we have looked at the hearts of some of the greatest Thoroughbreds and Quarter Horses around today. In his more than 20 years of measuring hearts, Dr. Fred Fregin has also compiled quite a record of what a truly great heart looks like, including that of the legendary Northern Dancer.

We thought it would be instructive for our readers to be able to see the actual ECGs of some of these great hearts, including such horses as champions John Henry, Alysheba, Cigar, Key to the Mint, and Holy Bull. We present these hearts on the following pages as an illustration of what is truly a "great heart" in a racehorse.

Alysheba • 1984

Alydar x Bel Sheba

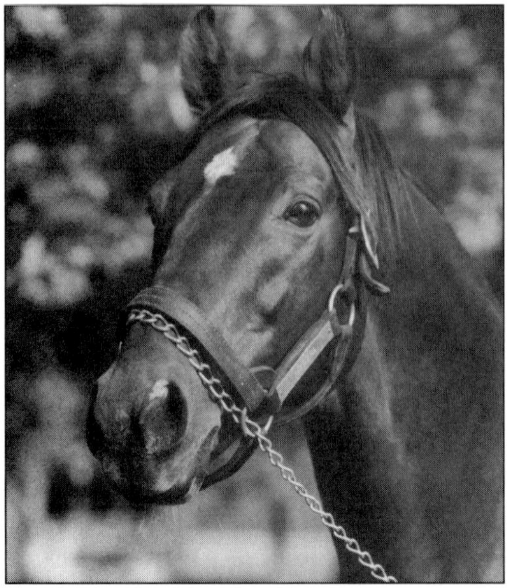

Photo courtesy of Patricia McQueen

Heart Score: 147

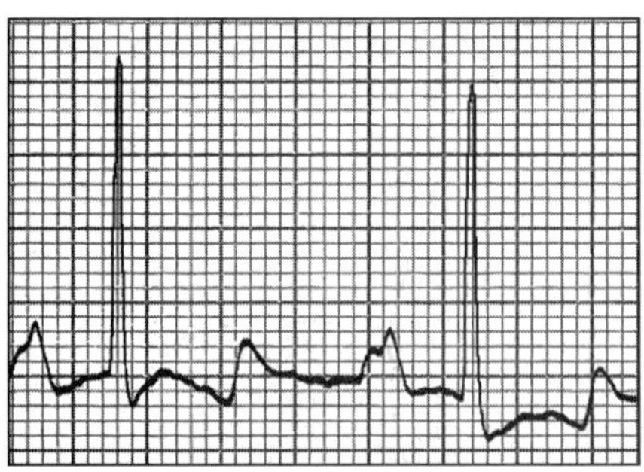

Race Record

	Starts	1st	2nd	3rd	Money Earned
Totals	26	11	8	2	$6,679,242

Bonnie's Poker • 1982

Poker x What A Surprise

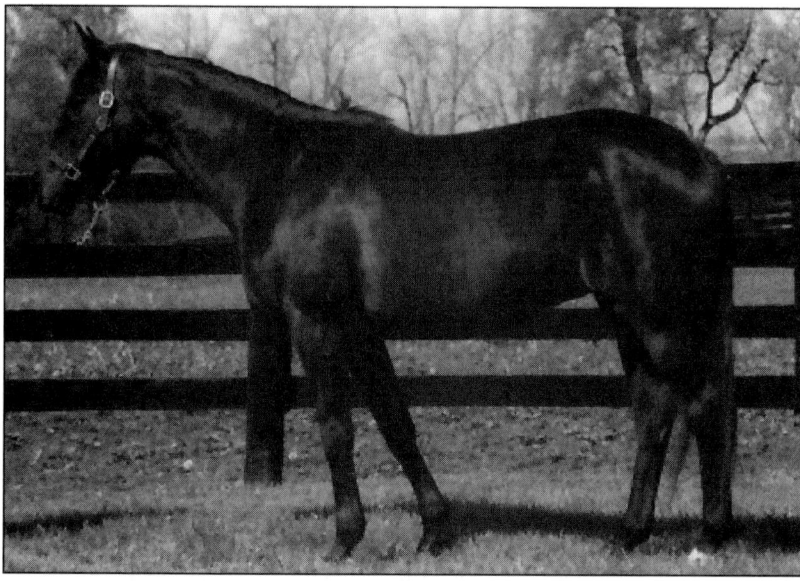

Photo courtesy of Kristi Jakeman

Heart Score: 147

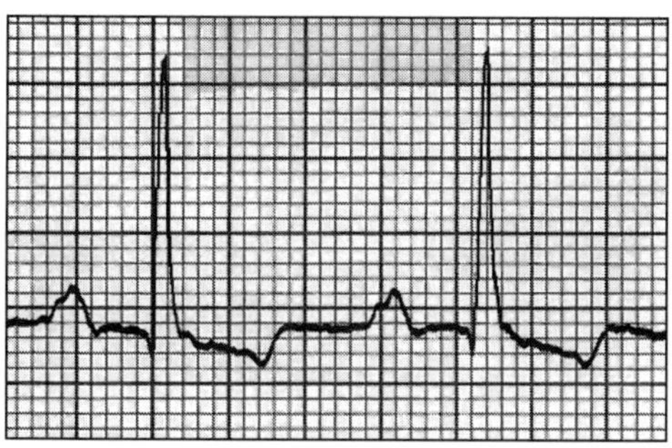

Race Record

	Starts	1st	2nd	3rd	Money Earned
Totals	63	11	9	10	$153,960

Cigar • 1990

Palace Music x Solar Slew

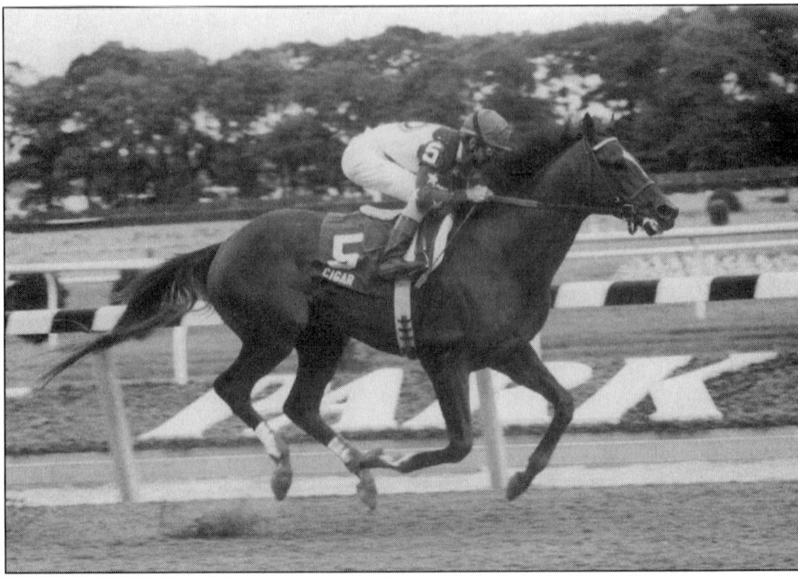

Photo courtesy of Patricia McQueen

Heart Score: 147

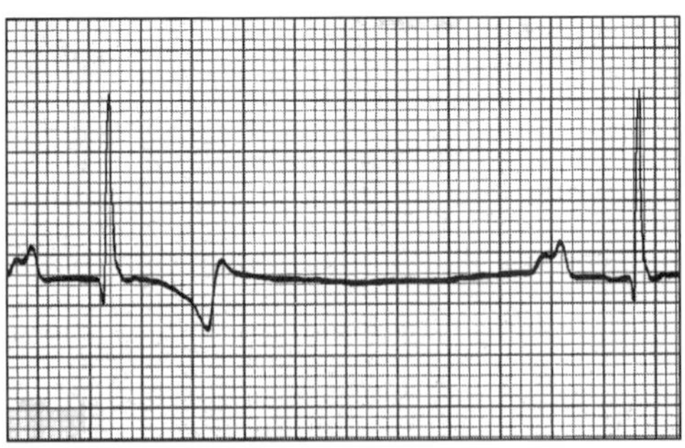

Race Record

	Starts	1st	2nd	3rd	Money Earned
Totals	32	18	4	5	$7,599,813

Corona Kool • 1997

First Down Dash x Sizzling Lil

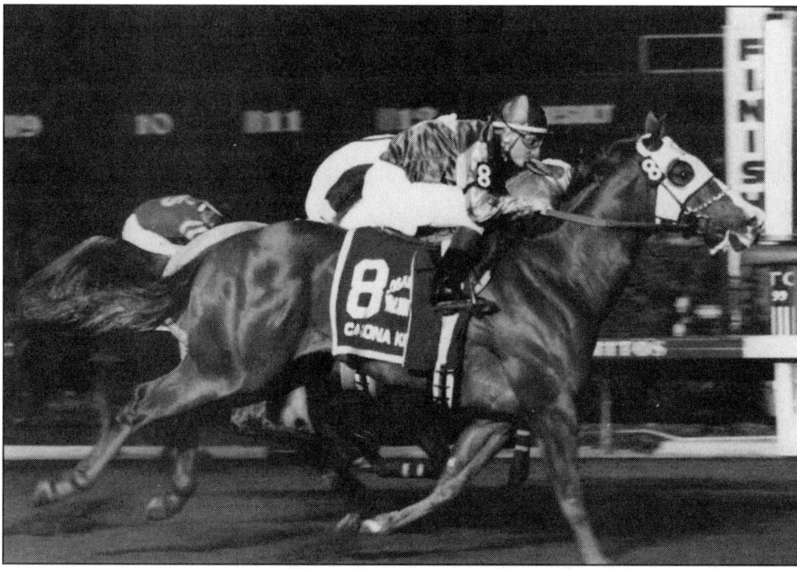

Photo courtesy of Scott Martinez/American Quarter Horse Journal

Heart Score: 130

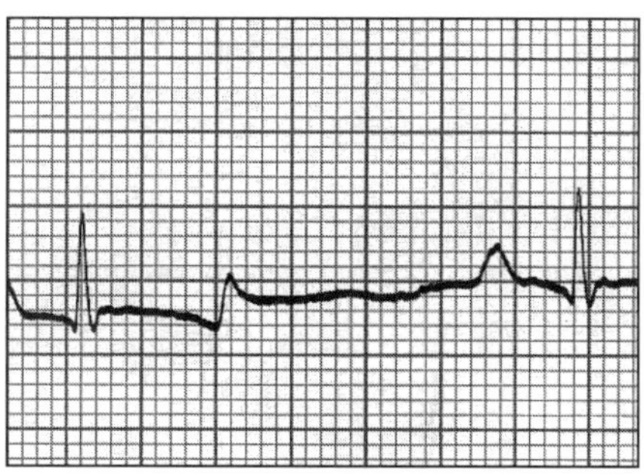

Race Record

	Starts	1st	2nd	3rd	Money Earned
Totals	22	12	3	3	$1,175,375

El Gran Senor • 1981

Northern Dancer x Sex Appeal

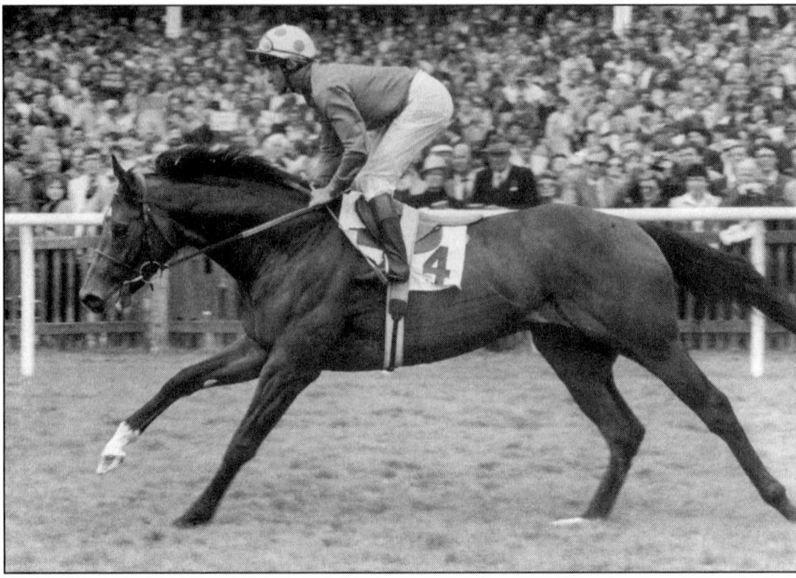

Photo courtesy of the Thoroughbred Times

Heart Score: 147

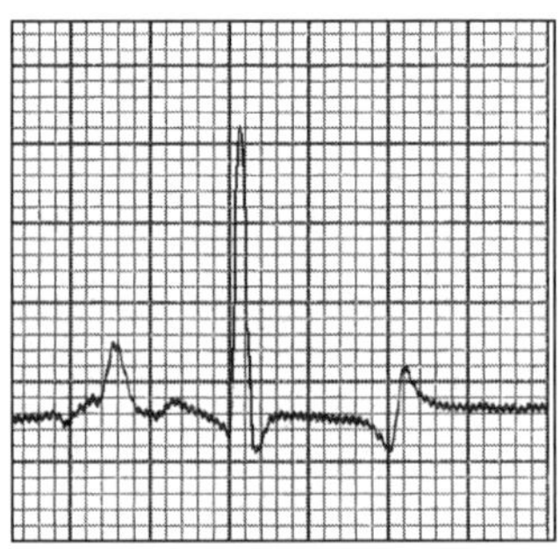

Race Record

	Starts	1st	2nd	3rd	Money Earned
Totals	8	7	1	0	$509,479

First Down Dash • 1984

Dash for Cash x First Prize Rose

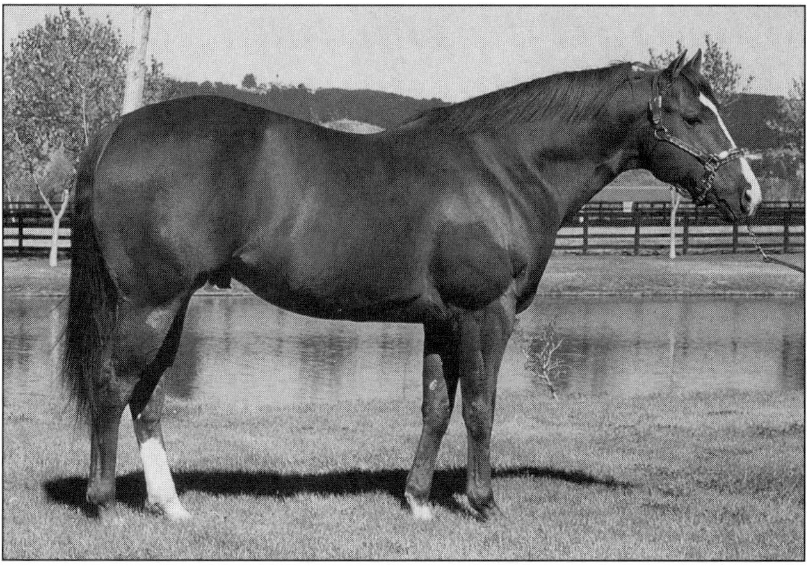

Photo courtesy of John Neal

Heart Score: 130

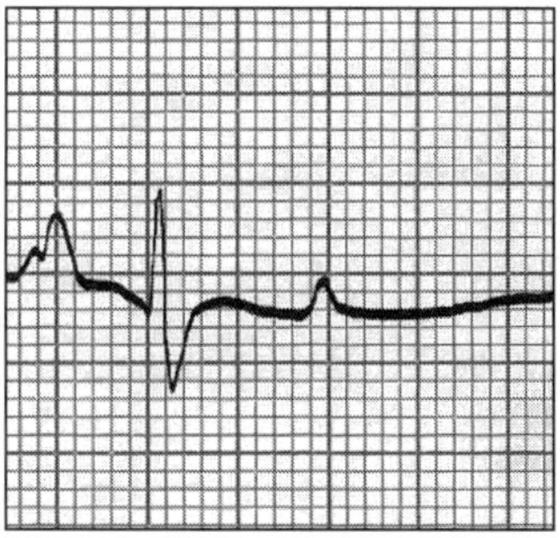

Race Record

	Starts	1st	2nd	3rd	Money Earned
Totals	15	13	1	0	$857,256

Holy Bull • 1991

Great Above x Sharon Brown

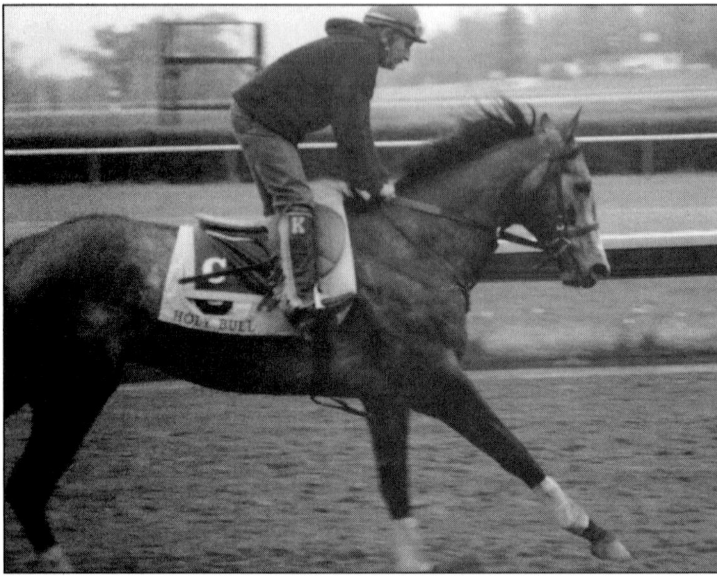

Photo courtesy of Marianna Haun

Heart Score: 147

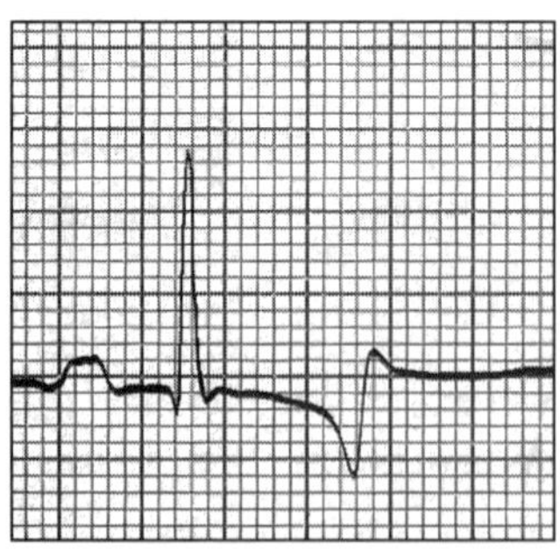

Race Record

	Starts	1st	2nd	3rd	Money Earned
Totals	16	13	0	0	$2,481,760

Huddle Up • 1982

Sir Ivor x Huggle Duggle

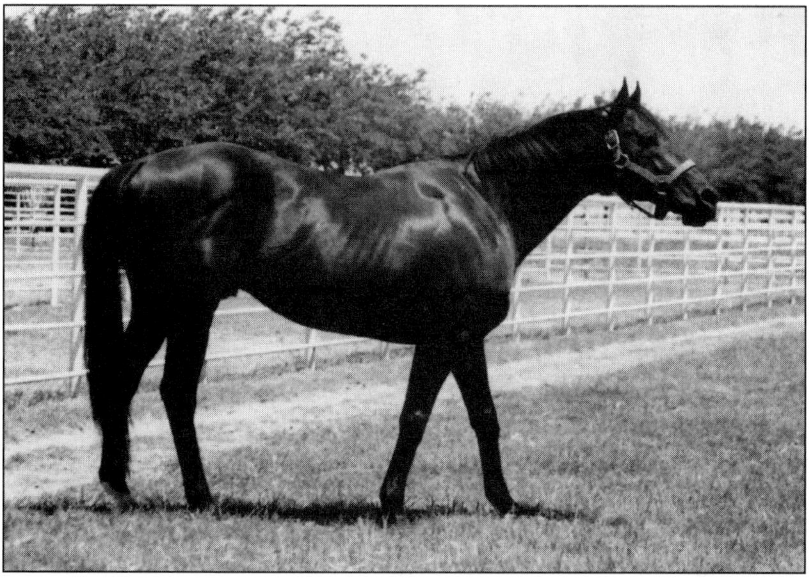

Photo courtesy of Marianna Haun

Heart Score: 147-150

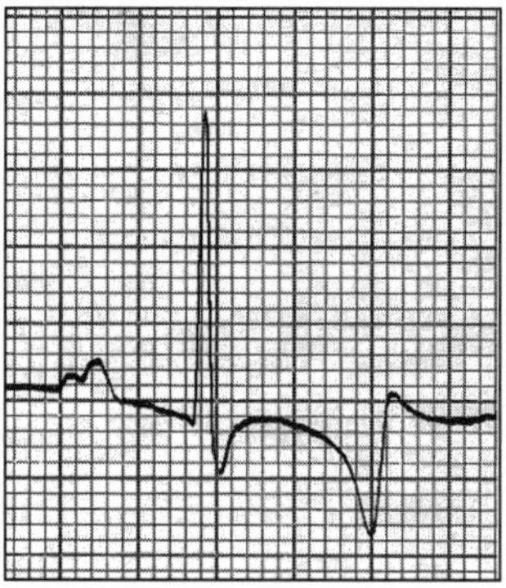

Race Record

	Starts	1st	2nd	3rd	Money Earned
Totals	16	3	2	5	$87,017

John Henry • 1975

Ole Bob Bowers x Once Double

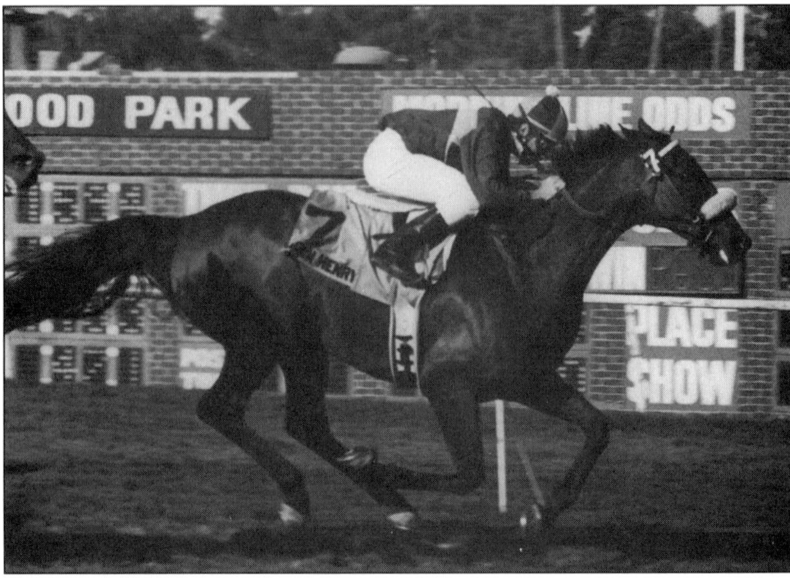

Photo courtesy of the Thoroughbred Times

Heart Score: 147

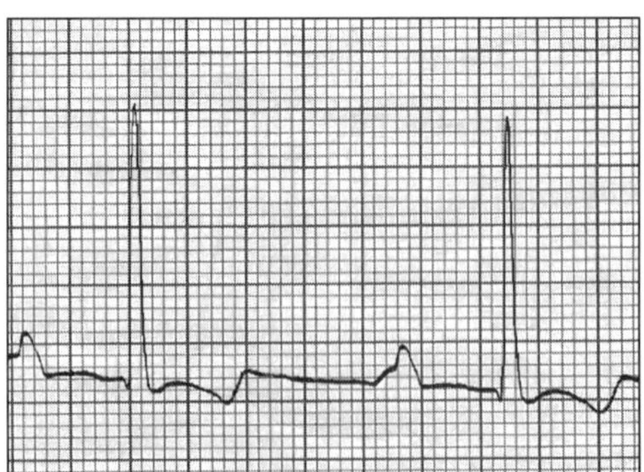

Race Record

	Starts	1st	2nd	3rd	Money Earned
Totals	82	39	15	9	$6,591,860

Key To The Mint • 1969

Graustark x Key Bridge

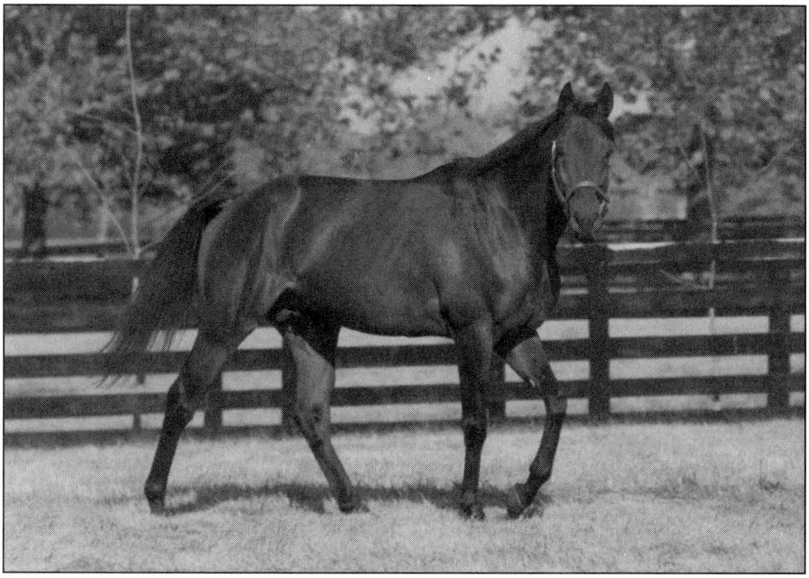

Photo courtesy of the Thoroughbred Times

Heart Score: 157-160

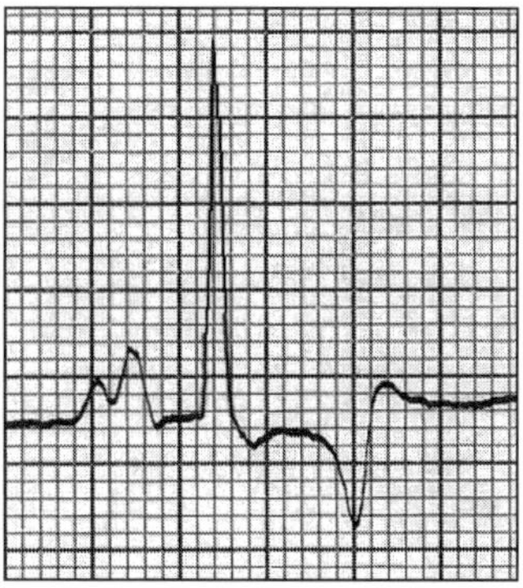

Race Record

	Starts	1st	2nd	3rd	Money Earned
Totals	29	14	4	3	$576,015

Lac Ouimet • 1983

Pleasant Colony x Northern Sunset

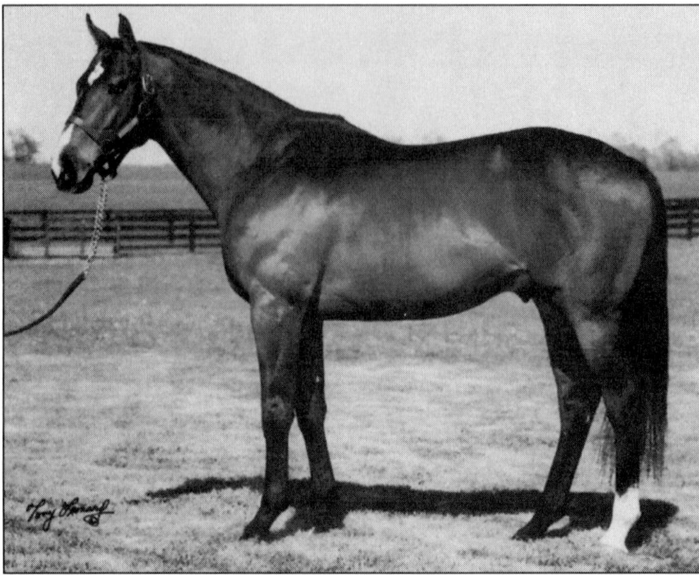

Photo courtesy of Tony Leonard

Heart Score: 140

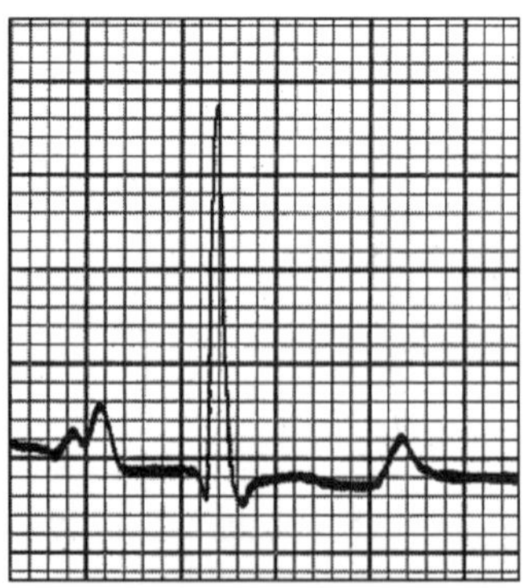

Race Record

	Starts	1st	2nd	3rd	Money Earned
Totals	40	12	8	3	$817,863

Moscow Ballet • 1982

Nijinsky II x Millicent

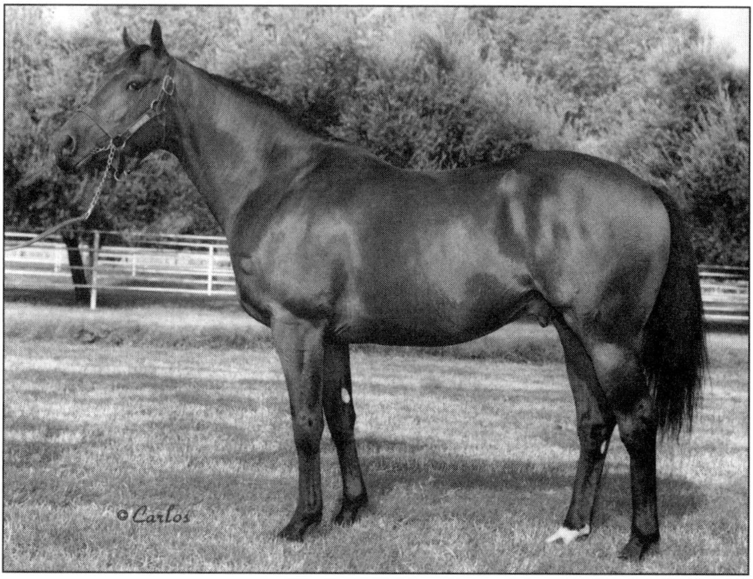

Photo courtesy of Mari Carlos

Heart Score: 147

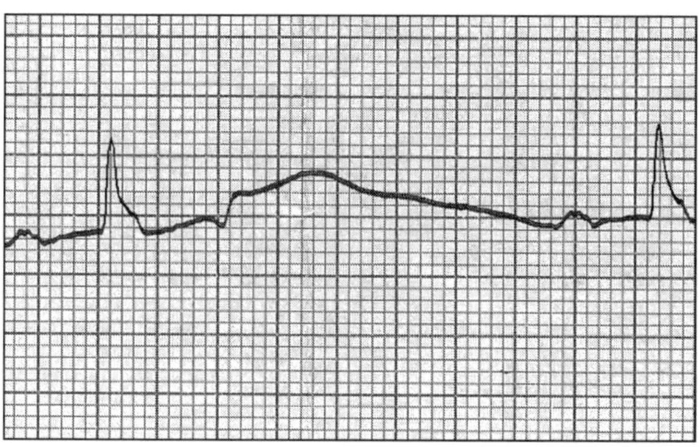

Race Record

	Starts	1st	2nd	3rd	Money Earned
Totals	4	2	0	0	$15,087

Northern Dancer • 1961

Nearctic x Natalma

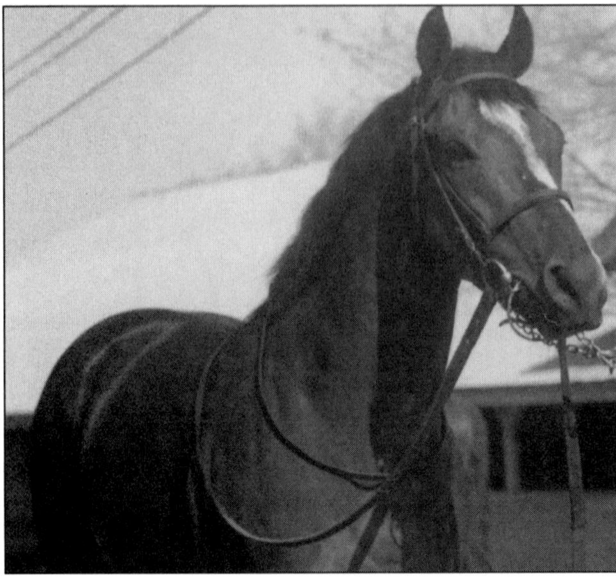

Photo courtesy of the Thoroughbred Times

Heart Score: 150

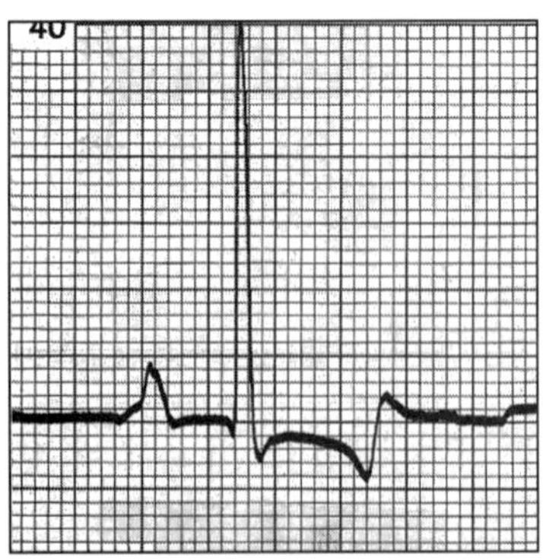

Race Record

	Starts	1st	2nd	3rd	Money Earned
Totals	18	14	2	2	$580,647

Northern Sunset • 1977

Northfields x Moss Greine

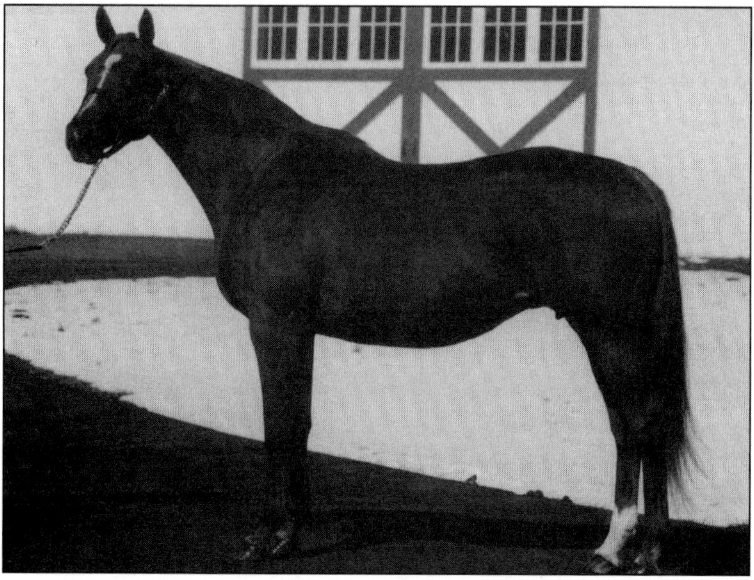

Photo courtesy of Laura Tucker, the Thoroughbred Times

Heart Score: 140

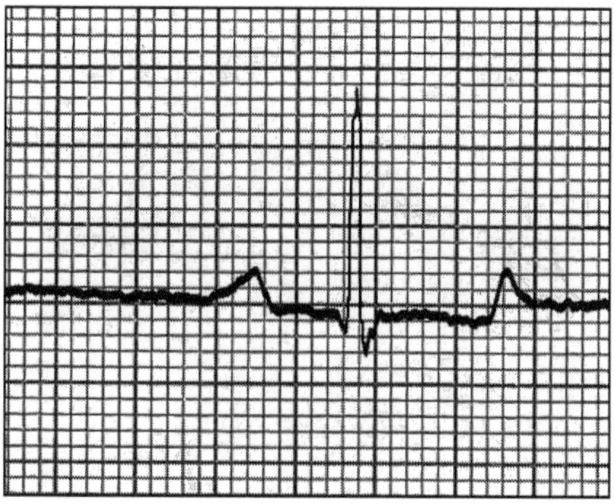

Race Record

	Starts	1st	2nd	3rd	Money Earned
Totals	16	2	4	0	$3,804

Private Account • 1976

Damascus x Numbered Account

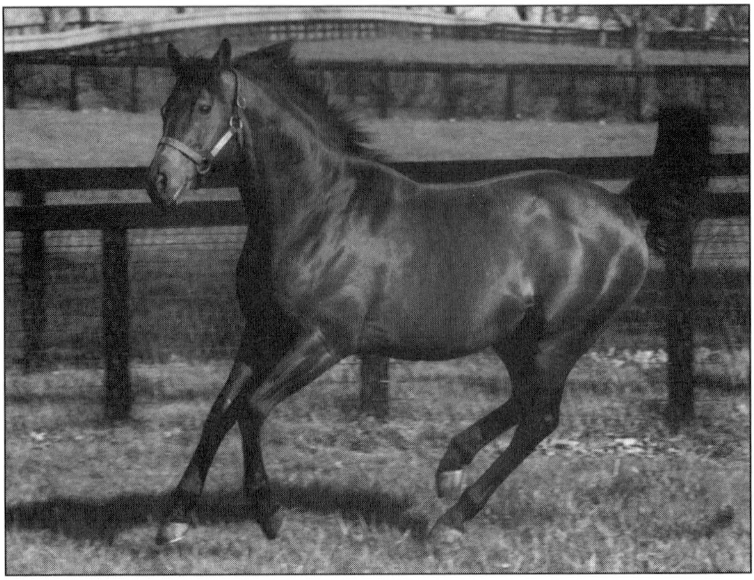

Photo courtesy of the Thoroughbred Times

Heart Score: 143

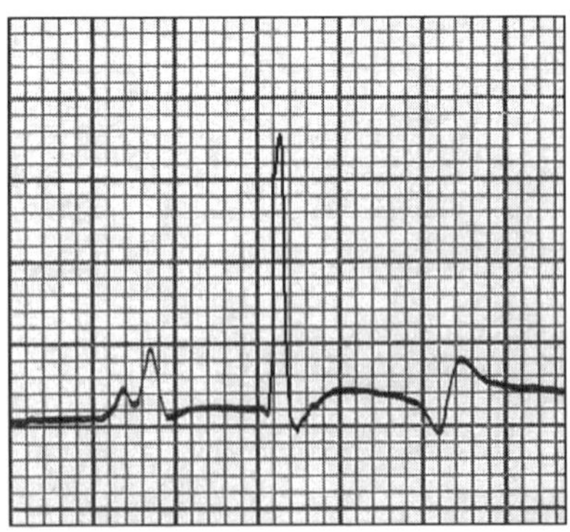

Race Record

	Starts	1st	2nd	3rd	Money Earned
Totals	13	6	4	1	$339,396

Pure D Dash

Dash for Cash x Native Noblesse

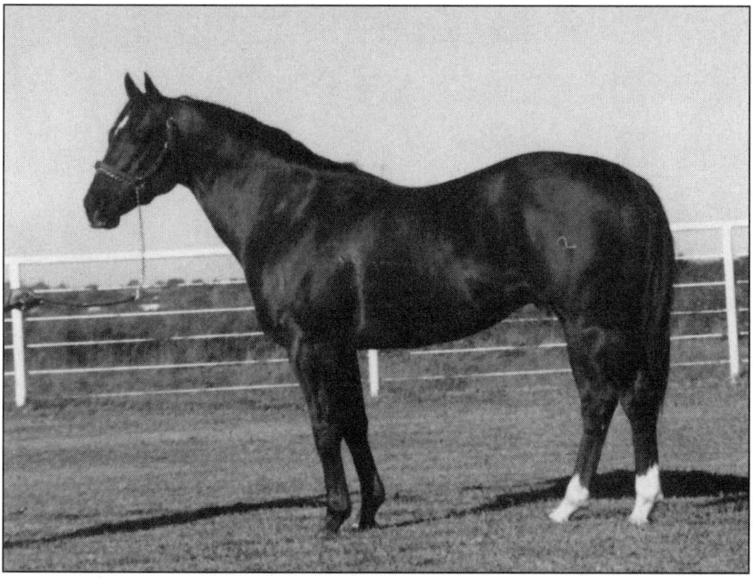

Photo courtesy of the Roy Browning Ranch

Heart Score: 130

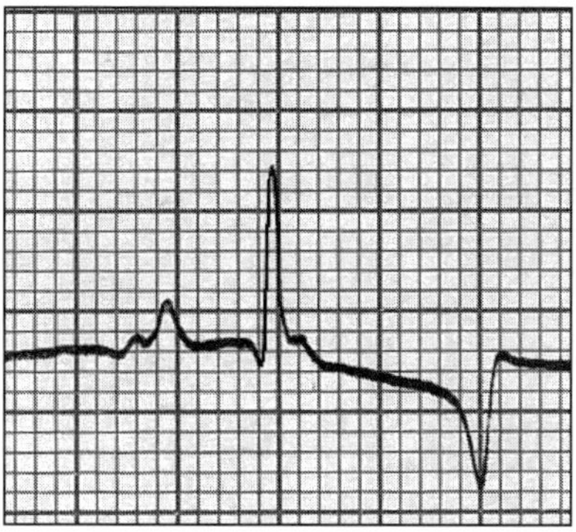

Race Record

	Starts	1st	2nd	3rd	Money Earned
Totals	27	7	5	4	$50,577

Pure Profit • 1983

Key To The Mint x Clear Ceiling

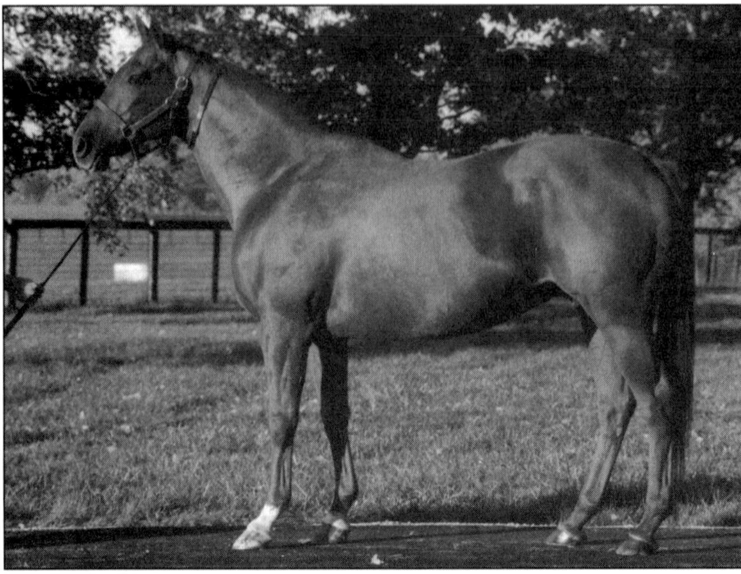

Photo courtesy of the Thoroughbred Times

Heart Score: 157

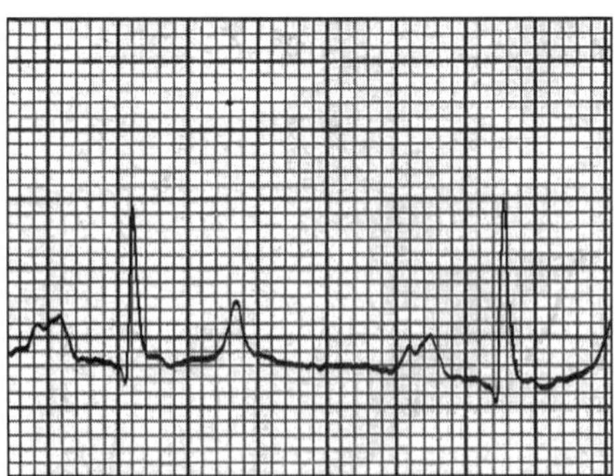

Race Record

	Starts	1st	2nd	3rd	Money Earned
Totals	5	4	0	1	$55,080

Rare Form

The Signature x Especially For You

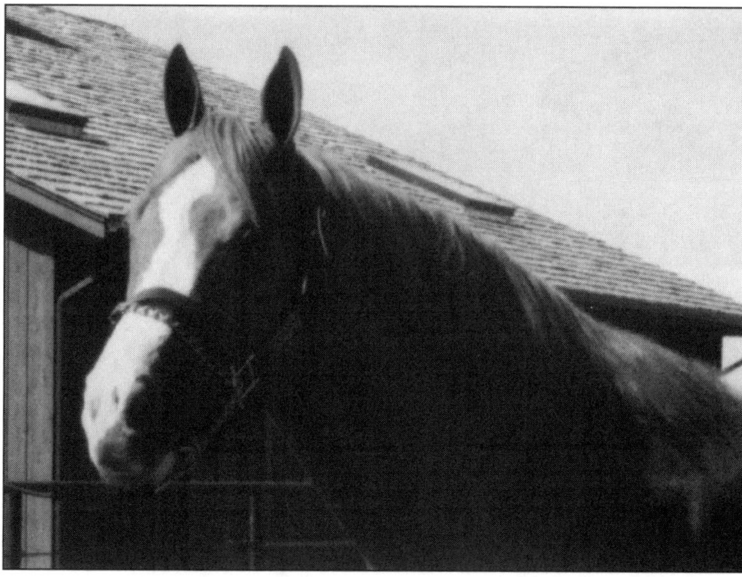

Photo courtesy of Amy Owens

Heart Score: 130

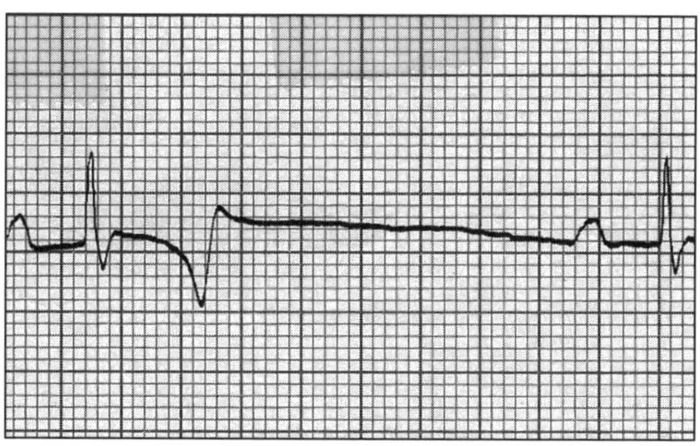

Race Record

	Starts	1st	2nd	3rd	Money Earned
Totals	27	17	2	2	$278,191

Salem Drive • 1982

Darby Creek Road x Northern Sunset

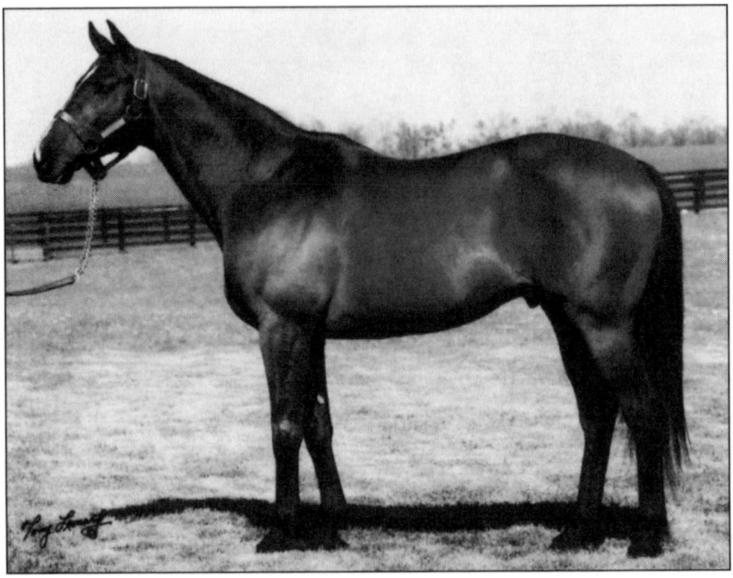

Photo courtesy of Tony Leonard

Heart Score: 140

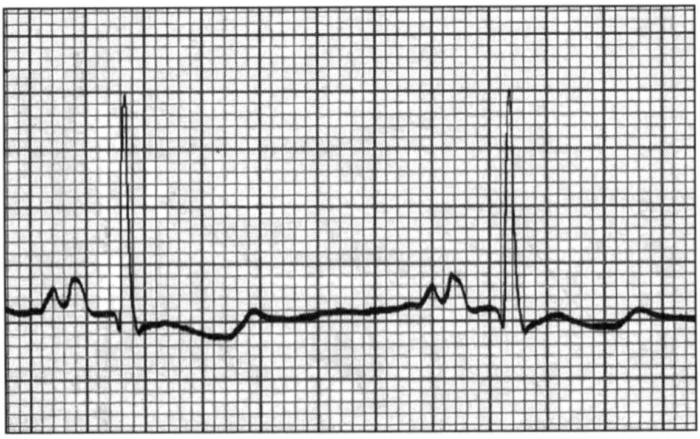

Race Record

	Starts	1st	2nd	3rd	Money Earned
Totals	46	13	7	10	$1,045,575

Sgt. Pepper Feature • 1970

Truckle Feature x Marketina

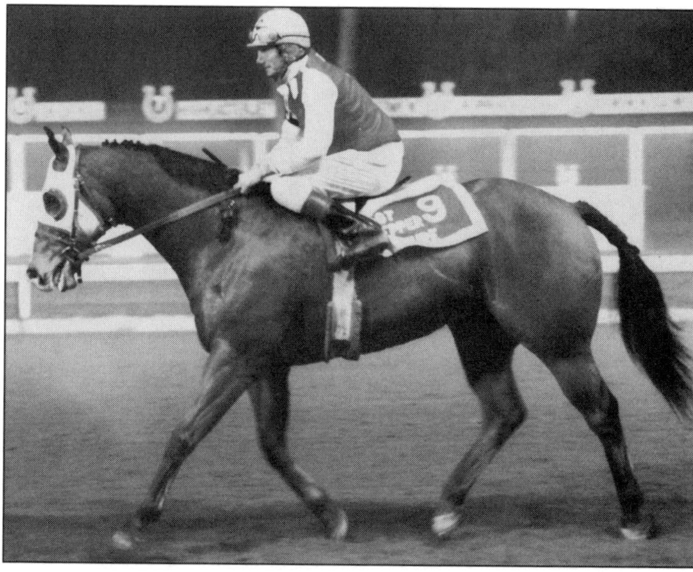

Photo courtesy of the Quarter Horse Racing Journal

Heart Score: 143

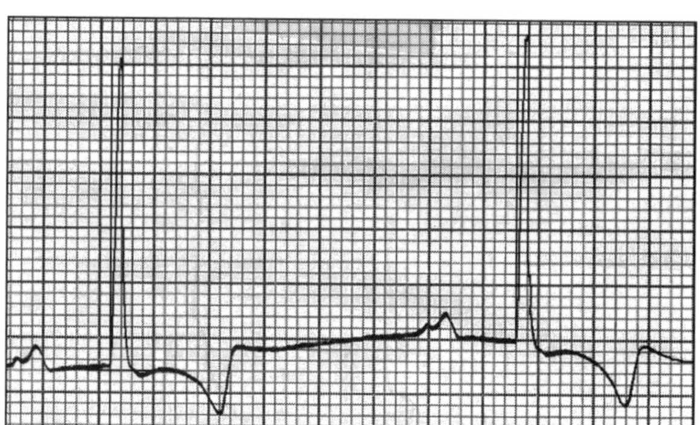

Race Record

	Starts	1st	2nd	3rd	Money Earned
Totals	62	20	11	8	$900,237

St. Jovite • 1989

Pleasant Colony x Northern Sunset

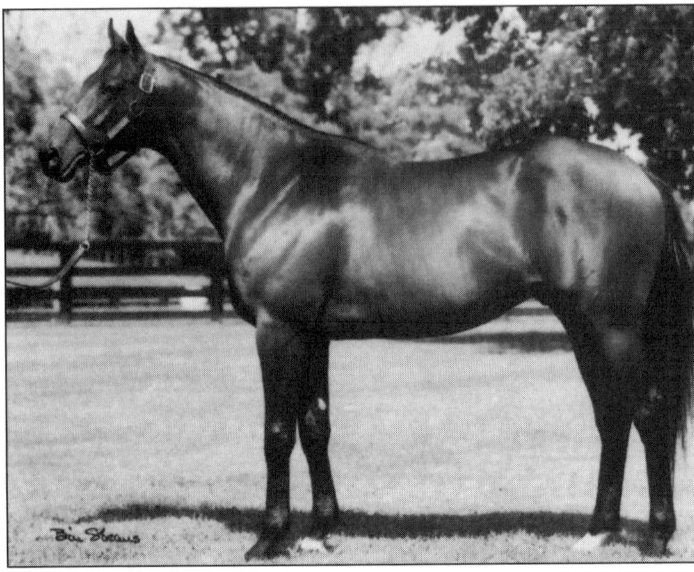

Photo courtesy of Tony Leonard

Heart Score: 140

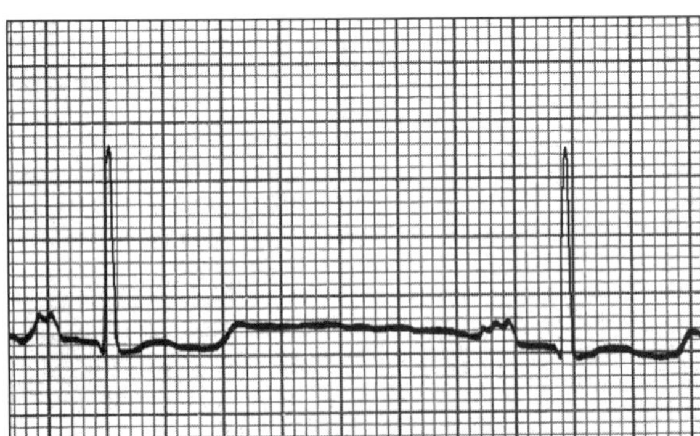

Race Record

	Starts	1st	2nd	3rd	Money Earned
Totals	11	6	2	0	$1,631,032

Weekend Surprise • 1980

Secretariat x Lassie Dear

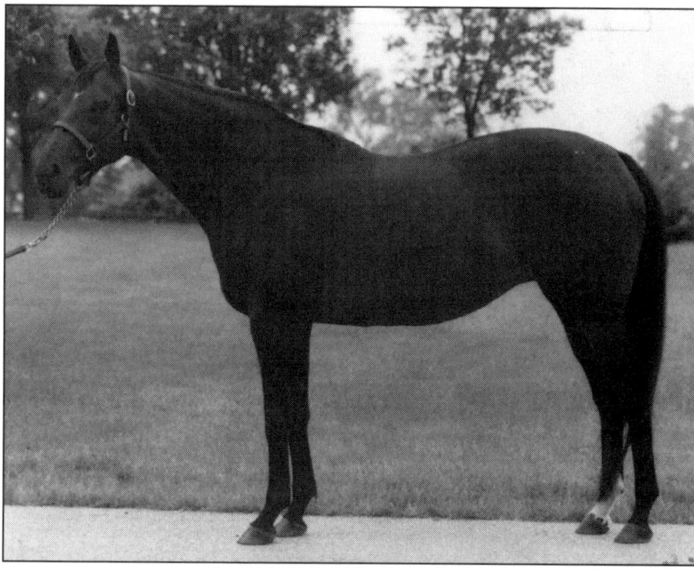

Photo courtesy of Photos by Z

Heart Score: 137

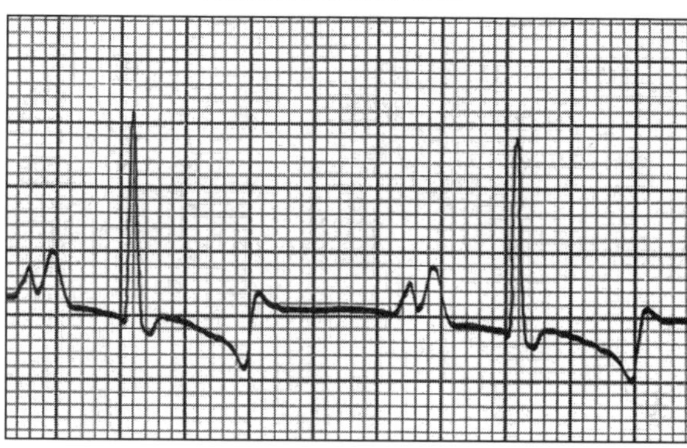

Race Record

	Starts	1st	2nd	3rd	Money Earned
Totals	31	7	5	10	$402,892

Woodman • 1983

Mr. Prospector x Playmate

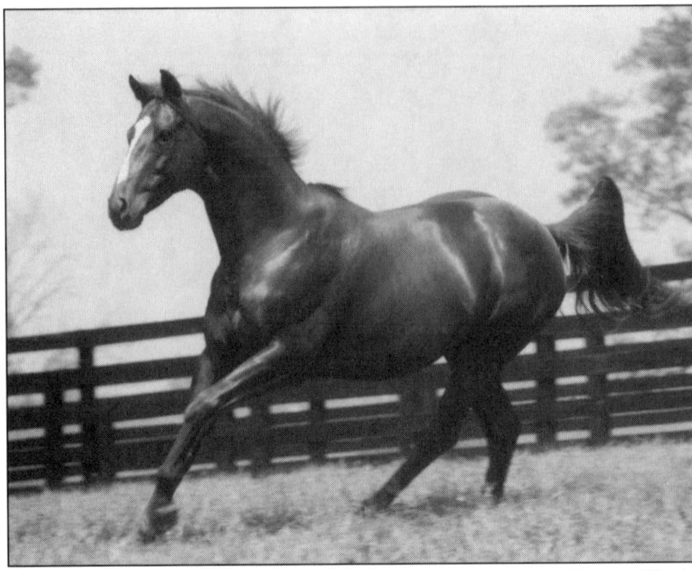

Photo courtesy of Photos by Z

Heart Score: 143

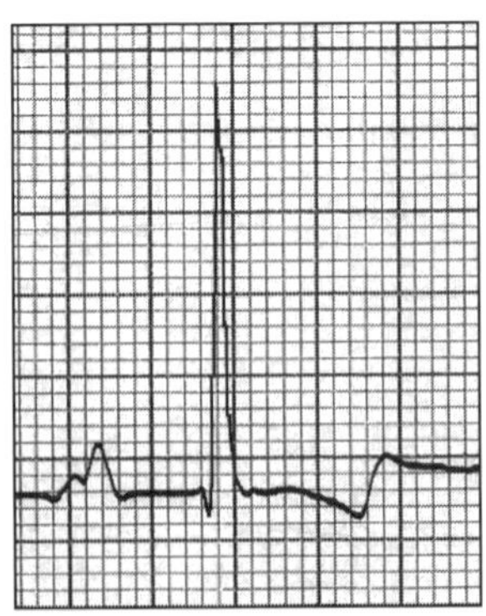

Race Record

	Starts	1st	2nd	3rd	Money Earned
Totals	5	3	0	1	$30,130

Index

Milan Mill, 59, 61, 107-108, 110, 112-113, 138, 141

Noble Victory, 152, 168-170, 173, 175